Curriculum for Culturally Responsive Health Care
The Step-By-Step Guide for Cultural Competence Training

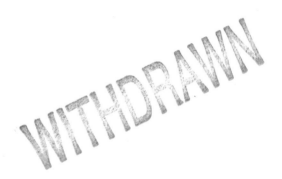

Curriculum for Culturally Responsive Health Care

The Step-By-Step Guide for Cultural Competence Training

JEFFREY M. RING, PhD, JULIE G. NYQUIST, PhD
SUZANNE MITCHELL, MD, HECTOR FLORES, MD,
and LUIS SAMANIEGO, MD

Family Medicine Residency Training Program
White Memorial Medical Center, Los Angeles

Radcliffe Publishing
Oxford • New York

Radcliffe Publishing Ltd
18 Marcham Road
Abingdon
Oxon OX14 1AA
United Kingdom

www.radcliffe-oxford.com
Electronic catalogue and worldwide online ordering facility.

British Library Cataloguing in Publication Data

A catalogue record for this book is available from the British Library.

ISBN-13: 978 184619 294 4

Typeset by Pindar NZ, Auckland, New Zealand
Printed and bound by Cadmus Communications, USA

Contents

Section 1

Introductory Materials

Acknowledgements

This curriculum was developed thanks to a generous grant and ongoing encouragement from the California Endowment, in particular Robert Ross, MD, Ignatius Bau, JD, and Jae Lee Wong.

Luis Guevara, PsyD and Elisa Munoz provided important contributions and support to the early development of the manuscript. Further, we could not have completed this project without the assistance of the staff of the Family Medicine Residency Office under the direction of Erasmo Cortez and Stephanie Gates.

We are grateful to our panel of community advisors who provided essential feedback during the early stages of development of the project, including:

Chungsheng Bai, PhD
David Chernof, MD
Patrick Dowling, MD
Jean Gilbert, PhD
David Hayes-Bautista, PhD
Luis Mata, MHA
Delight Satter, MPH
Kumea Shorter-Gooden, PhD
Beatriz Solis, MPH

A special expression of appreciation is due to the residents and faculty of the White Memorial Medical Center, Family Medicine Residency Training Program for their eagerness to participate in and provide feedback on all stages and aspects of this curriculum.

About the Authors

Jeffrey M. Ring, PhD is the Director of Behavioral Sciences at the White Memorial Family Medicine Residency Program in Los Angeles, where he teaches cultural medicine, doctor-patient communication, and mind-body medicine. He received his PhD in clinical psychology and is a Fellow of the Society for the Study of Ethnic Minority Issues (Division 45) of the American Psychological Association. Dr Ring is past Chair of the Society of Teachers of Family Medicine Group on Minority Health and Multicultural Education, and has led numerous workshops on culturally responsive medicine. He is the author of *The Long and Winding Road: Personal Reflections of an Anti-Racism Trainer* published in the American Journal of Orthopsychiatry.

Julie G. Nyquist, PhD is a Professor in the Division of Medical Education at the University of Southern California. She joined the faculty in 1981, directs the Master of Academic Medicine, and has specialized expertise in evaluation and faculty development. Dr Nyquist has given over 250 workshops, nationally and internationally, to faculty members from a variety of health professions. From 1993 to 2001 she also served as the Director of Medical Education at Kern Medical Center in Bakersfield, California, where she provided oversight for all educational activities (undergraduate, graduate, CME, and faculty development) within the medical center. Professor Nyquist received her doctorate in Educational Psychology from Michigan State University in 1981.

Dr Suzanne Mitchell, MD is a board certified family physician, medical educator, and consultant in cross-cultural medical care and communications. Dr Mitchell received her doctorate degree from the Wake Forest University School of Medicine and completed post-graduate training in Family Medicine at the White Memorial Medical Center Family Medicine Residency Program. Dr Mitchell also received a Masters of Science in Clinical Research from the University of California, Los Angeles and has engaged in health disparities research in the area of childhood obesity. Dr Mitchell resides in Massachusetts and holds faculty appointments at Harvard Medical School and Tufts University School of Medicine.

Dr Hector Flores , MD grew up in southern California and graduated from Stanford University with a BA in History. He attended the UC Davis School of Medicine and was honored with the Heineman Pulmonary Medicine Award and the Henry J. Kaiser Family Foundation National Fellowship. He completed his residency in Family Medicine at Kaiser Permanente in Los Angeles and is a founding member and Co-Director of the White Memorial Medical Center Family Medicine Residency Program. Dr Flores is the recipient of numerous academic and civic awards and in 2007 he received the Champions of Health Professions Diversity Award from The California Wellness Foundation.

Dr Luis Samaniego , MD was born and raised in Southern California. He obtained a BS Degree in Biology from Occidental College in 1977, received his medical degree from the University of Southern California in 1981 and went on to complete his internship and residency at Kaiser Permanente in Los Angeles. As a founding member of the White Memorial Medical Center Family Medicine Residency Program, he is completing his 20th year as residency director. Dr Samaniego also serves as President of the Family Care Specialists Medical Corporation.

Curriculum Preface

This curriculum has grown out of a long-term commitment to teaching culturally responsive medicine at the White Memorial Family Medicine Residency Program, working towards the elimination of health disparities, be they related to gender, race/ethnicity, income, sexual orientation, religious background or world view. The program, situated in a medically underserved, predominantly Latino community in East Los Angeles, was developed with the vision of training physicians who will be prepared to provide excellent, culturally and linguistically relevant medical care to patients.

In 2000, the California Endowment provided grant funding to formally put into operation, describe, enhance, and study the effects of our residency curriculum in culturally responsive medicine. This provided us with the support and opportunity to do the painstaking work of enhancing our pre-existing curriculum, interweaving it with the Accreditation Council for Graduate Medical Education (ACGME) and Association of American Medical Colleges (AAMC) requirements for medical education in culture, with attention to Culturally and Linguistically Appropriate Services (CLAS) Standards.

Our goal in this project was to produce a state-of-the art curriculum, with a manual that is creative, comprehensive, and user-friendly. The curriculum is intended for use by residencies, medical schools and other health professions' schools looking to implement new or enhance existing curricula in culturally responsive care. Furthermore, our aim has been to meticulously describe teaching strategies that will prove engaging to learners and faculty alike, challenging them to grow in their attitudes/awareness, desire, knowledge, and skills to effectively practice culturally responsive medicine. This is a curriculum that does not shy away from addressing the grueling social realities and oppression that form the foundation for ethnic/racial health disparities in the United States.

Our internal evaluation of the impact of the curriculum on our program and residents has revealed a growing impact in the following areas: a) places within the residency that are seen by residents as addressing the cultural competence objectives, b) consistently high rating of resident performance by peers, faculty, and patients in the area of professionalism, communication skills, and cultural competence, c) consistent perception by graduating residents that they have had the opportunity to master the awareness, knowledge, and skills objectives in the curriculum, d) increasing confidence in residents in their skills as they progress through the curriculum, and e) increased depth of insights seen in reflective writing.

It would be naïve to think that this curriculum is complete. There is no such thing as a static curriculum in an area so quickly shifting as the field of culturally responsive medicine. We are on the cusp of many new discoveries and potential ethical challenges associated with ethnic pharmacology, the genome project, and shifting demographics in this country. We hope this curriculum provides at least a solid foundation upon which educational programs can build as they evolve to meet the needs of patients and their communities toward preventing and treating illness, and improving access to excellence in medical care.

JMR, JGN, SM, HF, and LS
June 2008

How to Use This Curriculum

The reader is encouraged to tailor this curriculum to the unique requirements of the setting where cultural medicine will be taught. Our vision is that instructors will personalize sessions, modify them, implement them, and perhaps mix things up according to their own personal teaching style and institutional needs. The curriculum is organized into seven sections.

Section 1   Introductory Materials
Section 2   Overview of the Curriculum
Section 3   Step-by-Step Session Descriptions and Instructions
Section 4   Teaching Techniques
Section 5   Cultural Exercises
Section 6   Evaluation Tools
Section 7   Resources and References

Design (Sections 1 and 2)

This curriculum has been designed as a three-year, 33-hour, longitudinal curriculum in cultural competence and culturally responsive medicine. The instructional units and learning objectives are linked to the core competencies delineated by the ACGME (at www.acgme.org) and the AAMC as reflected in the Tool for Assessing Cultural Competence Training (TACCT at http://www.aamc.org/meded/tacct/culturalcomped.pdf). At the conclusion of training, learners will have received ample training and experience in the awareness/attitudes, knowledge, and skills components of culturally responsive care. Learning institutions that implement the curriculum should have an easy time preparing documentation of compliance with ACGME and AAMC requirements.

The curricular units parallel those in the AAMC document Cultural Competence Education for Medical Students (2005) and are listed below.

Unit I   Introduction to Culture and Cultural Competence (includes AAMC Domain I)
Unit II   Key Concepts in Cultural Competence (includes AAMC Domain II except community-related objectives)
Unit III   Bias, Stereotyping, Culture and Clinical Decision-Making (includes AAMC Domain III)
Unit IV   Health and Healthcare Disparities (includes AAMC Domain IV, except IVE)
Unit V   Cultural Competence in Patient Care (includes AAMC Domain V)
Unit VI   Cultural Competence and Community Action (includes AAMC Domain IVE)

Implementation in Residency Programs

The curriculum is designed for use during three years of a residency program. The curriculum is like an ever-spinning carousel. Riders can get on or off at any time, but as long as they stay three years, they will receive the entire training. The six units provide an organizing structure for the learning objectives. Objectives from every unit are addressed in each of the three years of the curriculum.

Given the rotation of residents into and out of training each year, the curriculum begins with three introductory overview sessions (Sessions A, B, and C) which can be presented as part of the intern orientation (a necessary initial introduction before getting on the ride). These sessions provide learners with the basics necessary to 'join in' with the three-year curriculum already in progress for the second and third year residents. As such, all residents will receive all three years of training, but in a different order of presentation, depending on their year in training.

The annual 10-session program follows the following agenda:

Sessions A, B, C   Introduction to basic concepts
Session 1   Bias, power and the doctor–patient relationship
Session 2   Effective communication – Part I

Session 3	Cultural knowledge of selected cultural groups
Session 4	Socio-cultural and political aspects
Session 5	Special populations
Session 6	Effective communication – Part II
Session 7	Cultural issues in teaching and research
Session 8	Annual review of health disparity data – selected topics
Session 9	Resident case presentations
Session 10	Annual review of progress

These are parallel, but not repeating, annual cycles. For example, the content for Session 1 each year is novel yet reinforces the learning of previous Session 1 material.

Implementation in Health Sciences Programs or Medical Institutions

Programs may desire greater flexibility in selecting topics and sessions for weekly courses or more compact intensive training workshops. For example, an instructor may want to structure a course according to the six AAMC Domains. Either way, this curriculum allows instructors to easily pick and choose learning activities when constructing their own educational plan for their learners.

Step-by-Step Session Descriptions and Teaching Methods (Section 3)

Each of the 33 sessions is described in great detail to aid the facilitator in preparing to teach. These teaching guides include a session description, a list of session objectives, and instructional materials required to run the session. This is followed by a time schedule for the (one hour) session. Specific instructions for teaching each component of the session are detailed in the Process section. As needed, additional cautionary notes are included at the end along with resources. Session timing is approximate. Instructors should never feel compelled to complete all activities, sometimes 'less is more'.

The teaching sessions have been designed to stimulate self-reflection, provoke new thinking, and facilitate the development of new clinical skills. Teaching activities range from interactive exercises to creative writing. There are video vignettes to stimulate discussion and role play exercises to practice interviewing strategies. Throughout the curriculum, learners will be asked to document their learning and to make commitments to their own application of new learning in the clinical setting.

Teaching Techniques (Section 4)

The next section of the curriculum contains detailed descriptions of commonly used teaching strategies that appear regularly throughout the 33 sessions. These have been divided into the following five categories.
1. Attention grabbers – activities that stimulate students' curiosity and involvement in the learning process.
2. Skill builders – activities that provide tangible hands-on experience in developing the awareness, knowledge, and skills necessary for culturally responsive care.
3. Catalysts – activities that stimulate learners to interact with the concepts presented and/or with each other.
4. Intensifiers – activities that deepen the learning in a very personal way, and promote positive, personal, professional development.
5. Trackers – techniques for charting learners' progress through the curriculum.

Cultural Exercises (Section 5)

Our program incorporates a variety of online, community-based, and classroom exercises, which are described here. Many of these are independent study activities that extend cultural medicine learning opportunities beyond the standard 'one-hour' format. Suggestions and guidelines for these exercises are included in this part of the curriculum handbook.

Tools (Section 6)

Here educators will find a growing set of tools that can be used to help teach and assess learners, as well as assist in the program evaluation. These include a Cultural Medicine Questionnaire, Commitment to Change forms and an example of a journal called a *Passport*. Each tool provides a different perspective and methodology for a) assessing a learner's progress through the curriculum in terms of awareness/attitudes, knowledge, and skills, or b) assessing or tracking the curriculum and the integration of concepts into the overall training program.

Resources and References (Section 7)

While each of the 33 sessions includes specific bibliography materials and ordering information for videos or other materials, this final section of the curriculum notebook includes website descriptions, information on selected video resources, books, and key journal articles for developing, extending, and deepening learning in culturally responsive care and cultural competence.

Concluding Thoughts

It is not easy to be a teacher. It is extremely challenging to shape a new generation of healers with an eye to excellence in care for all patients and the elimination of health and health care disparities. Socrates said, 'Education is the kindling of the flame, not the filling of a vessel.' In a sense, this curriculum is about kindling that flame in our learners toward the incineration of racism and other oppressions that continue to challenge the fields of health and medicine. Our development of this curriculum is one response to help others advance their teaching in this essential field. We welcome your enthusiasm, creativity, commitment, and feedback to the task at hand.

Section 2

Overview of the Curriculum

Curricular Units and Objectives

The following table describes the curriculum by unit and objective with the relevant objectives from the AAMC Tool for Assessment of Cultural Competence Training (TACCT), the relevant ACGME competencies, and the numbers of relevant curricular sessions noted. The right-most column indicates where each of the objectives is presented in our curriculum. Each objective includes a reference to key areas of emphasis: A = awareness/attitudes; K = knowledge; Sk = skills; PBLI = practice-based learning and improvement; I&CS = interpersonal and communication skills.

Curricular Units and Objectives

Unit	No.	Objectives	AAMC Objectives	ACGME Competencies	Session Numbers
Unit I Introduction to Culture and Cultural Competence (includes AAMC Domain I)	1	Define, in contemporary terms, race, ethnicity, and culture, and their implications in health care (K)	IK1	Knowledge	A, 1, 11
	2	Become aware of their own cultural heritage, gender, class, ethnic/racial identity, sexual orientation, disability, age, and spirituality; be able to reflect on it and describe it (A, Sk)	IA1, ISII, IIIS4	Professionalism	B, 10, 20, 30
	3	Value the importance of diversity in health care and address the challenges and opportunities it poses (A)	IA3	Professionalism	A, C, 3, 13, 14, 23
	4	Identify patterns of national data on health, health care disparities, and quality of health care, and be able to discuss (K)	IK3, IK4	Knowledge	8, 18, 28
	5	Discuss the epidemiology of health and health care disparities for the local community using *Healthy People 2010* and other resources (K, Sk)	IS3, IIIS6, IVK4	Knowledge, PBLI	8, 18, 28
Unit II Key Concepts in Cultural Competence (includes AAMC Domain II except community-related objectives)	6	Value the importance of social determinants (e.g. education, culture, socioeconomic status, housing, and employment) and community factors on health and strive to address them (A, Sk)	IIA3	Systems-based practice	C, 24
	7	Describe historical models of common health beliefs (e.g. illness in the context of 'hot and cold') and identify questions about health practices and beliefs that might be important in a specific local community (K)	IIK1, VK1	Patient care	3, 9, 13, 19, 23, 29
	8	Identify healing traditions and beliefs of patients and/or their families, including ethno-medical beliefs. Ask questions in a non-judgmental manner to elicit patient preferences, listen and respond appropriately to patient feedback about key cross-cultural issues. Elicit additional information about ethno-medical conditions and ethno-medical healers (A, K, Sk)	IIK2, IIS2, IIA2	Patient care, I&CS	B, 6, 9, 12, 19, 29
	9	Discuss race, ethnicity, and culture in the context of the medical interview and health care. Exhibit comfort when conversing with patients/colleagues about cultural issues (A, Sk)	IIS3, IIA1	Patient care, I&CS	B, 3, 7, 12, 13, 17, 23
	10	Recognize and describe institutional cultural issues for own institution; discuss CLAS Standards (Sk)	IIS5	Systems-based practice	14, 22
	11	Value the importance of curiosity, empathy, and respect in patient care and the importance of continuous growth as a healer (A)	IIA4	Professionalism	7, 17, 27

cont.

Unit	No.	Objectives	AAMC Objectives	ACGME Competencies	Session Numbers
Unit III Bias, Stereotyping, Culture and Clinical Decision-Making (includes AAMC Domain III)	12	Recognize their own potential for bias and stereotyping, be able to identify their own stereotypes and biases and explore how their attitudes, biases and stereotypes affect clinical encounters, clinical decision-making, and quality of care (A, K)	IIIK3, IIIA1, IIIA3, IIIA4, VA2	Professionalism, patient care	1, 10, 11, 20, 21, 30
	13	Identify and appreciate how clinician bias and stereotyping can affect interactions with patients, families, communities, and other members of the health care team, and the link between effective communication and quality care (A, K)	IA2, IIIK2, IIIA2	Professionalism, I&CS	1, 11
	14	Describe the impact of the patient's context (cultural heritage, gender, class, ethnic-racial identity, sexual orientation, disability, age and spirituality) on clinical decision-making (K)	IIIK1	Knowledge	7, 17
	15	Describe strategies for reducing physician's own biases, and those of others and demonstrate strategies to assess, manage, and reduce bias and its effects in the clinical encounter and in clinical practice (Sk)	IIIS1, S2, S3, IVS4, VS5	Patient care, PBLI	10, 20, 21, 30
	16	Describe the inherent power imbalance between physician and patient and how it affects the clinical encounter (K)	IIIK4	I&CS	21
Unit IV Health and Healthcare Disparities (includes AAMC Domain IV, except E)	17	Recognize and describe how access, historical, political, environmental, and institutional factors (including racism and discrimination) impact health and underlie health and health care disparities (A, K)	IVK1, IVA2	Knowledge	4, 5, 15, 25
	18	Identify how race, ethnicity and social determinants of health (e.g. education, culture, socioeconomic status, housing and employment) affect health and health care quality, cost, and outcomes (K)	IVK2	Knowledge	4, 5, 15, 25
	19	Identify and discuss the contributors to disparities (patient, provider, health care system, and society) and discuss the challenges and barriers to eliminating health disparities (K)	IVK4, IVK6	Knowledge	4, 24, 25
	20	Describe patterns of health care disparities that can result, at least in part, from clinician bias, recognize disparities that are amenable to intervention, and value eliminating disparities (A, K)	IIIK5, IVA1, IVA3	Professionalism, systems-based practice	4, 5, 10, 15, 20, 25, 30
	21	Describe systemic and medical-encounter issues related to health care disparities, including communication issues, clinical decision-making, and patient preferences (K)	IVK3	I&CS	5, 11, 14, 15
Unit V Cultural Competence in Patient Care (includes AAMC Domain V)	22	Describe models of effective cross-cultural communication, assessment, and clinician–patient negotiation and identify common challenges in cross-cultural communication (for example, trust, style) (K)	IIK3, VK2, VK3	I&CS	2, 9, 16, 19, 26, 29
	23	Conduct and document a culturally responsive history and physical examination within the context of family-centered care. Elicit a cultural, social, and medical history, including a patient's health beliefs/model of their illness. Demonstrate respect for patients' cultural and health beliefs and use negotiating and problem-solving skills in shared decision-making with a patient (A, Sk)	IS1, VS1, VS2, VA1	Patient care, professionalism I&CS	2, 12, 16, 22, 26
	24	Describe the functions of an interpreter and effective ways of working with an interpreter. Identify when an interpreter is needed and collaborate effectively with an interpreter (K, Sk)	VK4, VK5, VS3	I&CS	22
	25	Assess and enhance patient adherence based on the patient's explanatory model. Describe ways to enhance patient adherence by collaborating with traditional/community healers (K, Sk)	VK6, VS4	I&CS, patient care	6, 9, 19, 26, 29

cont.

Unit	No.	Objectives	AAMC Objectives	ACGME Competencies	Session Numbers
Unit V (*cont.*)	26	Critically appraise the literature as it relates to health disparities, including systems issues and quality in health care (Sk)	IVS1	PBLI	8, 18, 28
Unit VI Cultural Competence and	27	Describe factors that contribute to variability in population health; outline a framework to assess communities according to population health criteria, social mores, cultural beliefs, and needs (K, Sk)	IIK6, IIS1	PBLI, systems-based practice	C
Community Action (includes AAMC Domain IVE)	28	Describe methods to identify key community leaders. Describe strategies for partnering with community activists to eliminate racism and other bias from health care. Develop a proposal for a community-based health intervention. Collaborate to address community needs (K, Sk)	IVS2, IIS4, IVS3, IIIK6	Systems-based practice	3, 13, 23, 24

Resource

Healthy People 2010. Available from: http://www.healthypeople.gov/Document/tableofcontents.htm

Theoretical Basis for Selection of Objectives and Activities

The following table describes four theoretical/developmental perspectives that guided the authors in the development of content and activities within the curriculum. This is a practical manual, and thus the theory underlying the materials is not brought into the actual curricular sessions.

TABLE 2.1 Theoretical Basis for Selection of Objectives and Activities

Carrillo *et al.*, 1999[1]	Wells, 2000[3]	Camphina-Bacote, 2002[4]	AAMC, 2005[5]
Module 1. **Basic concepts**: definition of culture	**Cultural awareness**: recognizing and understanding the cultural implications of behavior	**Cultural awareness**: the self-examination and in-depth exploration of one's own cultural and professional background	Domain I. **Cultural competence – rationale, context, and definition**: understanding importance of cultural competence and relationship with health disparities, defining terms, individual self-assessment of own culture and bias
Module 2. **Core cultural issues**: situations, interactions, and behaviors that have potential for cross-cultural misunderstanding	**Cultural knowledge**: Learning the elements of culture and their role in shaping and defining health behavior	**Cultural knowledge**: the process of seeking and obtaining a sound educational foundation about diverse cultural and ethnic groups, including health-related beliefs and cultural values, disease incidence and prevalence, and treatment efficacy	Domain II. **Key aspects of cultural competence**: population health, patient/family-centered care, institutional cultural issues, patient and community
Module 3. **Understanding the meaning of the illness**: using Kleinman's questions with patients – patient's explanatory model[2]	**Cultural sensitivity**: the integration of cultural knowledge and awareness into individual and institutional behavior	**Cultural skill**: the ability to collect relevant cultural data regarding the client's presenting problem as well as accurately performing a culturally based physical assessment	Domain III. **Understanding the impact of stereotyping on medical decision-making**: bias, stereotyping, discrimination, racism, impact on clinical decision-making
Module 4. **Determining the patient's social context**: clinicians learn practical techniques to explore and manage the social factors most relevant to the medical encounter	**Cultural competence**: the routine application of culturally appropriate health care	**Cultural encounters**: cultural encounter is the process that encourages the health care provider to directly engage in cross-cultural interactions with clients from culturally diverse backgrounds	Domain IV. **Health disparities and factors influencing health**: history of discrimination, epidemiology and patterns of health and health care disparities, factors underlying disparities, collaborating to eliminating disparities
Module 5. **Negotiating across cultures**: six phases – relationship building, agenda setting, assessment, problem clarification, management, and closure	**Cultural proficiency**: the integration of cultural competence into one's repertoire for scholarship	**Cultural desire**: the motivation of the health care provider to *want* to, rather than *have* to, engage in becoming culturally aware, knowledgeable, skillful, and familiar with cultural encounters	Domain V. **Cross-cultural clinical skills**: knowledge, respect, validation of difference, all skills needed to gather data, communicate, negotiate, diagnose, manage, and promote adherence

References

1. Carrillo JE, Green AR, Betancourt JR. Cross-Cultural Primary Care: A patient-based approach. *Ann Intern Med.* 1999; **130**(10): 829–34.
2. Kleinman A, Eisenberg L, Good B. Culture, illness, and care: clinical lessons from anthropologic and cross-cultural research. *Ann Intern Med.* 1978; **88**: 251–8.
3. Wells MI. Beyond cultural competence: a model for individual and institutional cultural development. *J Community Health Nurs.* 2000 Winter; **17**(4): 189–99.
4. Camphina-Bacote J. The process of cultural competence in the delivery of healthcare services: a model of care. *J Transcult Nurs.* 2002 Jul; **13**(3): 181–4.
5. Association of American Medical Colleges. *Cultural Competence Education for Medical Students: Assessing and Revising Curriculum.* Washington D.C., 2005. Available from: http://www.aamc.org/meded/tacct/start.htm

Resources: Training Programs in Cultural Competence, Theory and Practice

Anderson LM, Scrimshaw SC, Fullilove MT, *et al.* Task Force on Community Preventive Services. Culturally competent healthcare systems: a systematic review. *Am J Prev Med.* 2003 Apr; **24**(3 Suppl.): 68–79.

Berlin FA, Fowkes Jr WC. A teaching framework for cross-cultural health care: application in family practice. *West J Med.* 1983; **139**: 934–8.

Betancourt JR. Cultural competence and medical education: many names, many perspectives, one goal. *Acad Med.* 2006 Jun; **81**(6): 499–501.

Betancourt JR, Green AR, Carrillo JE, *et al.* Defining cultural competence: a practical framework for addressing racial/ethnic disparities in health and health care. *Public Health Rep.* 2003 Jul–Aug; **118**(4): 293–302.

Crandall SJ, George G, Marion GS, *et al.* Applying theory to the design of cultural competency training for medical students: a case study. *Acad Med.* 2003 Jun; **78**(6): 588–94.

Culhane-Pera K, Like R, Lebensohn-Chialvo P, *et al.* Multicultural curricula in family practice residencies. *Family Med.* 2000; **32**(3): 167–73.

Ferguson WJ, Keller DM, Haley HL, *et al.* Developing culturally competent community faculty: a model program. *Acad Med.* 2003 Dec; **78**(12): 1221–8.

Hobgood C, Sawning S, Bowen J, *et al.* Teaching culturally appropriate care: a review of educational models and methods. *Acad Emerg Med.* 2006; **13**: 1288–95.

Kripalani S, Bussey-Jones J, Katz MG, *et al.* A prescription for cultural competence in medical education. *J Gen Intern Med.* 2006 Oct; **21**(10): 1116–20.

Lewis-Fernandez R, Diaz N. The cultural formulation: a method for assessing cultural factors affecting the clinical encounter. *Psychiatr Q.* 2002; **73**(4): 271–95.

Purnell L. The Purnell Model for cultural competence. *J Transcult Nurs.* 2002; **13**(3): 193–6.

Rust G, Kondwani K, Martinez R, *et al.* A crash-course in cultural competence. *Ethn Dis.* 2006; **16**(2 Suppl. 3): S29–36.

Thom DH, Tirado MD, Woon TL, *et al.* Development and evaluation of a cultural competency training curriculum. *BMC Med Educ.* 2006; **6**: 38.

Vega WA. Higher stakes ahead for cultural competence. *Gen Hosp Psychiatry.* 2005 Nov–Dec; **27**(6): 446–50.

Section 3

Step-By-Step Session Descriptions and Instructions

Curricular Sessions:
Overview and Table of Contents

Overview

Recall that Sessions A, B, and C are repeated each year during orientation to provide basic information for new residents. Sessions 1–10 are presented in Year 1, Sessions 11–20 in Year 2, and Sessions 21–30 in Year 3 of this spiral curriculum.

Table of Contents

cont.

SESSION A Introduction to Culture

Session Description

This first session takes place during orientation when most learners are still getting acquainted. This session is designed to introduce learners to each other and to the basic terms that underlie the entire cultural medicine curriculum (race, ethnicity, culture, diversity). The session begins by asking learners to fill out the Cultural Medicine Questionnaire (CMQ) as a baseline assessment of awareness and knowledge. A brief experiential exercise allows for an introductory exploration of similarities and differences. This is followed by a discussion of culture and its elements.

New in this session: This session introduces one tool, the CMQ, described in Section 6, and one method, 'debriefing', described in Section 4. If these are unfamiliar to you, you may wish to review the relevant entries.

Session Objectives

After participation in the session, learners should be better able to:
1. define, in contemporary terms, race, ethnicity, and culture and their implications in health care (Objective 1 – knowledge)
2. value the importance of diversity in health care and address the challenges and opportunities it poses (Objective 3 – attitudes).

Instructional Materials

Cultural Medicine Questionnaires; pens; glossary handout; flipcharts and markers.

Time Schedule

00:00 – 00:05   Session introduction
00:05 – 00:20   CMQ and discussion
00:20 – 00:30   2×2 exercise – similarities and differences
00:30 – 00:40   Debriefing 2×2 exercise
00:40 – 00:55   Interactive exercise
00:55 – 01:00   Session conclusion

Process

1. Session introduction (5 minutes): the session introduction serves as an opportunity to introduce presenter and participants, if they are not familiar to one another. The session objectives are presented, and an explanation given on how this session is an initial building block for the larger culturally responsive care curriculum.
2. CMQ and discussion (15 minutes): participants are provided copies of the CMQ and are asked to fill it out to the best of their ability. It is important to remind them that many of the questions do not necessarily have one correct answer. After collecting the CMQ there is a brief opening for discussion about it. Participants may have reactions and/or questions that the instructor(s) can address. If terms or concepts were not understood, these can be explained at this time.
3. 2×2 exercise – similarities and differences (10 minutes): this is a three-stage experiential exercise to facilitate exploration of human similarities and differences. First, ask participants to find a partner and introduce themselves (ideally a partner they do not know).
   - Task 1. Instruct the pairs to talk for three minutes and find as many similarities between them as possible (minimum of five). The only exception is that the similarities cannot have anything to do with medicine, the training program they are in, etc.
   - Task 2. At the conclusion of the three minutes, ask each pair to join with another pair, making groups of four (one group of six is alright if there is an uneven number of groups). The task for these new, larger groups is exactly the same: in three minutes find as many similarities as possible (still not related to medicine) between ALL of them.
   - Task 3. At the conclusion of the three minutes, ask each small group to break up into pairs again, but with someone they had not been originally paired with. This new pair

has the task to find as many differences between them as they can in three minutes, with a minimum of five.

4. Debriefing 2×2 exercise (10 minutes): the instructor can use the following series of questions with the whole group.
   - What are some examples of similarities identified in the first pairing?
   - What similarities were identified in the second small groups?
   - What strategies were used to find similarities in the small groups?
   - Did any groups encounter situations where all but one member shared a similarity? What was that like for the individual and the larger group?
   - What differences were identified in the final pairing?
   - Did you find that it was easier to identify similarities or differences? Why?
   - Did any of the groups explore any of the following as similarities or differences: religion, political party affiliation, gender, physical disability, race/ethnicity, or sexual orientation?

It is helpful to ask the group what they have surmised about the learning objectives of this exercise. Some of these are: team building, understanding more about the dynamics of similarities and differences, and the concept of 'comfort zones'. The group is encouraged to consider whether they are more comfortable with similarities or differences, and with which types of similarities and differences. Part of the challenge of becoming culturally responsive or culturally competent clinicians requires learners to stretch beyond their personal comfort zones and be able to comfortably interact and work with people who are both similar and markedly different.

5. Interactive exercise (15 minutes): ask the group to call out responses to the question: why has it become so important that health professionals learn to be culturally competent/culturally responsive? The instructor should capture these ideas on a master list on a flipchart at the front of the room. Some of the responses one might expect are as follows:
   - to be a better clinician
   - to better respond to changing demographics in the US
   - to improve patient satisfaction
   - to improve provider satisfaction
   - to enhance practice building
   - to decrease malpractice complaints
   - to eliminate health care disparities
   - social justice
   - Federal Standards (CLAS Standards)
   - insurance company (payor) audits of culturally and linguistically appropriate care.

A second question for brainstorming is to ask the group to define the word 'culture', capturing the elements of the definition suggested by the group on a flipchart at the front of the room.

Here is a definition of culture that can be shared with the group at the conclusion of the brainstorm session (perhaps handed out on a glossary page).

Culture is an integrated pattern of learned core values, beliefs, norms, behaviors and customs that are shared and transmitted by a specific group of people. Some aspects of culture, such as food, clothing and behavior, are visible. Major aspects of culture, such as values, gender role definitions, health beliefs and world view, are not visible.

6. Session conclusion (5 minutes): conclude with a review of the importance of the session's goals and central learning points. If you are with the group that will be working together throughout the full cultural competence curriculum, you might briefly introduce it here (2 minutes). For residents: 'The cultural competence curriculum will be woven throughout your three years of training. Each year you will have sessions related to expanding your awareness in relation to hidden bias; learn about and discuss health and health care disparities and their underlying causes; discuss various cultural groups and challenges related to effective care; have the opportunity to gain skills related to cultural competence and consider issues beyond your own care.'

Resources

Center for Health Equity Research and Promotion Collaborations: Glossary at Website http://www.cherp.org/introhd.php

Culhane-Pera K, Like R, Lebensohn-Chialvo P, *et al*. Multicultural curricula in family practice residencies. *Fam Med*. 2000; **32**(3): 167–73.

Fadiman A. *The Spirit Catches You and You Fall Down*. New York: Farrar, Straus, Giroux; 1998.

Kleinman A, Benson P. Anthropology in the clinic: the problem of cultural competency and how to fix it. *PLoS Med*. 2006 Oct; **3**(10): e294.

Kleinman A, Eisenberg L, Good B. Culture, illness, and care: clinical lessons from anthropologic and cross-cultural research. *Ann Intern Med*. 1978; **88**: 251–8.

Satcher D, Pamies R. *Multicultural Medicine and Health Disparities*. New York: McGraw Hill; 2006.

SESSION B Team Building: Awareness of Self and Others

Session Description
This session focuses on building a community of learners through enhanced understanding of self and others and is a basic building-block session for the entire curriculum. Learners explore the importance of personal story and the power of cultural context through use of a written autobiography (1 hour session) or a genogram (1 hour per learner).

Understanding your history and family dynamics is an essential component of becoming a compassionate, culturally responsive practitioner. Understanding your colleagues' cultural and family backgrounds can help build positive and empathic teams. This exercise is typically used as part of orientation when team-building is most crucial. Judgment forms quickly in terms of perceptions as to the nature and worthiness of any group experience. A good start sets the stage for everything that follows. The leaders of the cultural competence curriculum set the tone. Being approachable, warm, setting learners at ease and communicating excitement for the curriculum, and your role in it, is a good beginning. You want the learners to look forward to working together within the cultural competence curriculum.

At the end of this session, and most sessions throughout the curriculum, a technique called 'commitment to change' is used to encourage learners to take the new attitudes, knowledge and skills directly into their patient care settings, and to help them keep track of these 'promises' across time.

New in this session: This session introduces the autobiography or genogram exercise (if selected for use) described in Section 5, and the method, 'commitment to change' described in Section 4. If these are unfamiliar to you, please review the relevant entries.

Session Objectives
After participation in the session, learners should be better able to:
1. discuss his/her cultural heritage, gender, class, ethnic-racial identity, sexual orientation, disability, age, and spirituality; to reflect on it and describe it (Objective 2 – awareness)
2. identify healing traditions and beliefs, including ethno-medical beliefs of own family and those of peers (Objective 8 – attitude, skills)
3. exhibit comfort when conversing with colleagues about cultural issues (Objective 9 – attitude).

Instructional Materials
Instructions for autobiography (or genogram), distributed to learners approximately one week prior to the session; audiovisual equipment (if genograms are to be presented); index cards or prepared forms for commitment to change.

Time Schedule
00:00 – 00:10   Session introduction
00:10 – 00:50   Autobiography or genogram presentations
00:50 – 00:55   Commitment to change
00:55 – 01:00   Session conclusion

Process
Prior to Session
Provide learners with the autobiography assignment and explain that everything we do emanates from who we are (our personal wiring and our stories). Stories help us understand ourselves, and others. As part of building a community we will each write our story and share it with others in the group. Have learners submit their autobiographies in a timely manner, so that the lead faculty can read all of them prior to the session.

During the Session

1. Session introduction (10 minutes): this session is introduced with a brief review of the autobiography assignment and the instructor(s) briefly share their own story with the learners. Personal story is very powerful and setting the correct tone is important. The instructors should follow the directions provided in the autobiography entry in Section 5.
2. Autobiography or genogram presentations (40 minutes): if the group is small (5–8 people) try to schedule enough time so that everyone has a chance to share with the whole group. If the group is larger, typically you will need several groups. In the small groups, each person should have a minimum of 5 minutes to talk. Some groups may choose to make copies and share their written autobiographies with each other. The groups should be reminded to include information regarding their families' health practices and beliefs in their sharing.
3. Commitment to change (5 minutes): ask participants to make note (on index cards or on a form prepared for the session) what they will strive to do differently as a learner and physician, based on having prepared their own, and having listened to other learner's autobiographies.
4. Session conclusion: conclude with a review of the importance of the session's goals and central learning points. Invite learners to take new insights and knowledge directly back into their clinical work.

Resources

Boomer E, Reagan D, Galindo I. *A Family Genogram Workbook.* Nebraska: Educational Consultants; 2006. Available from: www.galindoconsultants.com

Campbell TL, McDaniel SH, Cole-Kelly K, *et al.* Family interviewing: a review of the literature in primary care. *Fam Med.* 2002 May; **34**(5): 312–8.

Kamei R. Professionalism: looking for your blind spots. *Ann Acad Med Singapore.* 2006; **35**(12): 848–84.

Sociology Central. *Genograms.* Available from: http://www.sociology.org.uk/as4fm3a.pdf

SESSION C Community Connections: Neighborhood Study

Session Description

This session is designed to help learners begin to connect with the community in which their patients live. Learners complete an independent study activity. They go in small groups (two to six learners) to visit a portion of the community surrounding the medical center in which they will be studying or working. The groups spend approximately one hour walking in the neighborhood following the directions provided in the assignment. Prior to debriefing, the learners produce a map, drawing, or photo collage showing what they saw and learned. During the debriefing, each of the groups shares their 'map' and discusses their experience. The session concludes with a reflective writing exercise.

New in this session: this session introduces the Neighborhood Study exercise described in Section 5 and two methods, independent study and reflective writing, described in Section 4.[1,2] If these are unfamiliar to you, please review the relevant entries.

Session Objectives

After participation in the session, learners should be better able to:
1. value the importance of diversity in health care and address the challenges and opportunities it poses (Objective 3 – attitudes)
2. value the importance of social determinants (e.g. education, culture, socioeconomic status, housing, and employment) and community factors on health and strive to address them (Objective 6 – attitudes)
3. describe factors that contribute to variability in population health; outline a framework to assess a community according to population health criteria, social mores, cultural beliefs and needs (Objective 27 – knowledge).

Instructional Materials

Neighborhood Study instructions; paper, markers, and other art supplies for each small group; maps of the neighborhood, one for each group, with their assigned area clearly highlighted.

Time Schedule

Option 1 – Products Made in Class

00:00 – 00:05	Session introduction and distribution of art supplies
00:05 – 00:30	Map/product preparation
00:30 – 00:50	Sharing of products and discussion of session objectives
00:50 – 01:00	Reflective writing and session conclusion

Option 2 – Products Brought to Class

00:00 – 00:05	Session introduction, paraphrasing of independent study assignment
00:05 – 00:30	Sharing of products and student insights into the community and the activity
00:30 – 00:50	Discussion of each of the factors listed on the Neighborhood Study exercise
00:50 – 01:00	Reflective writing and session conclusion

Process

Prior to Session

Independent study activity – the learners complete the Neighborhood Study, as instructed prior to coming to class.
1. Map out a section of the community surrounding the medical center and assign each pair/trio of students a segment that includes several residential and several non-residential blocks.
2. Provide instructions: 'You and your partner(s) will spend approximately one hour exploring the assigned community area and observing the aspects of community listed on your Neighborhood Study instructions. Your community survey will be enhanced if you are able to speak with members of the community (e.g. school teacher, local pharmacist, store

owner, priest, local clinic personnel, or people living in the community), shop at a store, or eat at a restaurant.'

3. If the learners are able to go as a group into the community just prior to your meeting, they can complete the map in class. Otherwise, they should complete it prior to class. Instructions: 'Prepare a product, a *Community Map* that captures the community. The product can be an actual hand-drawn map (with illustrations and labels), photo collage, poem, essay, etc. Please be as creative as you wish in drafting important features of your *Community Map*. Art supplies are available for your use. Be prepared to discuss your findings and your *Community Map* at our next meeting.'

During Session

1. Introduction (5 minutes): if the learners will be completing their maps in class, distribute the art supplies and get the groups started on their *Community Maps* or other creative projects. If they are bringing their products to class, the session could begin by paraphrasing the directions for the Neighborhood Study.

2. Option 1 – Product created in class
   a) Map/product preparation (25 minutes): as detailed in the assignment directions, learners are to prepare a map of the area visited using the flipchart paper and art supplies provided. This will be shared in the group presentations to follow.
   b) Small group presentations and discussion (20 minutes): time required will depend on the number of groups and the depth of the presentations. Each group shares their map, their observations of the people and community, and discusses community diversity, social determinants of health, and any factors that might contribute to variability in the health of groups in the community.

   Option 2 – Learners bring their completed projects to class
   a) Small group presentations and discussion (25 minutes): time required will depend on the number of groups and the depth of the presentations. Each group shares their map, their observations of the people and community, as well as risk factors (e.g. number of bars, graffiti, trash) and supportive factors (health clinics, natural healers, etc.).
   b) Discussion of each of the factors listed on the Neighborhood Study exercise (20 minutes): Each factor is related to the health risks and protective factors in the community as seen by the entire group. Challenge the students to outline elements of a framework that could be used to actually assess the community.

3. Reflective writing and session conclusion (10 minutes): participants are encouraged to write their reflections on the Neighborhood Study assignment and discussion – how it affected them, what feelings arose and how what they learned will affect their future practice/ learning of medicine with patients from this community. Their reflections can also be creative (using prose or poetry). Conclude with a brief review of the importance of the session's central learning points, inviting learners to take what they learned today directly back into their clinical work.

References

1. Eugenia E, Blanchard L. Action-oriented community diagnosis: a health education tool. *Int Q Community Health Educ.* 1991; **11**(2): 93–110.
2. Sloane P, Slatt L, Ebell M, *et al.* editors. *Essentials of Family Medicine.* Baltimore: Lippincott Williams & Wilkins; 2002.

Resources: Neighborhoods and Health

Browning CR, Cagney KA. Moving beyond poverty: neighborhood structure, social processes, and health. *J Health Soc Behav.* 2003 Dec; **44**(4): 552–71.

Eschbach K, Mahnken JD, Goodwin JS. Neighborhood composition and incidence of cancer among Hispanics in the United States. *Cancer.* 2005 Mar 1; **103**(5): 1036–44.

Hook EB. RE: 'Neighborhood social environment and risk of death: multilevel evidence from the Alameda County study'. *Am J Epidemiol.* 2000 Jun 1; **151**(11): 1132–3.

Lambert SF, Brown TL, Phillips CM, *et al.* The relationship between perceptions of neighborhood characteristics and substance use among urban African American adolescents. *Am J Community Psychol.* 2004 Dec; **34**(3–4): 205–18.

Lash TL, Fink AK. RE: 'Neighborhood environment and loss of physical function in older adults: evidence from the Alameda County Study'. *Am J Epidemiol.* 2003; **157**(5): 472–3.

Latkin CA, Curry AD. Stressful neighborhoods and depression: a prospective study of the impact of neighborhood disorder. *J Health Soc Behav*. 2003; **44**(1): 34–44.

Leventhal T, Brooks-Gunn J. Moving to opportunity: an experimental study of neighborhood effects on mental health. *Am J Pub Health*. 2003 Sep; **93**(9): 1576–82.

Nordstrom CK, Diez Roux AV, Jackson SA, *et al*. Cardiovascular Health Study. The association of personal and neighborhood socioeconomic indicators with subclinical cardiovascular disease in an elderly cohort. *Soc Sci Med*. 2004; **59**(10): 2139–47.

Pickett KE, Ahern JE, Selvin S, *et al*. Neighborhood socioeconomic status, maternal race and preterm delivery: a case-control study. *Ann Epidemiol*. 2002 Aug; **12**(6): 410–18.

Thompson DR, Iachan R, Overpeck M, *et al*. School connectedness in the health behavior in school-aged children study: the role of student, school, and school neighborhood characteristics. *J School Health*. 2006 Sep; **76**(7): 379–86.

Unnatural Causes Website http://www.unnaturalcauses.org

Willems S, Vanobbergen J, Martens L, *et al*. The independent impact of household- and neighborhood-based social determinants on early childhood caries: a cross-sectional study of inner-city children. *Family Community Health*. 2005 Apr–Jun; **28**(2): 168–75.

Yen IH, Kaplan GA. Neighborhood social environment and risk of death: multilevel evidence from the Alameda County Study. *Am J Epidemiol*. 1999; **149**(10): 898–907.

SESSION 1 Bias and Stereotyping

Session Description

This session focuses on the recognition of bias and its impact on health care quality. Learners are asked prior to the session to complete several Implicit Association Tests (IATs) online (*see* Implicit Association Test in Section 5 for details). The session opens with a debriefing of the exercises and a discussion of reactions and lessons learned. Within the session, the learners participate in an Imagery exercise that helps them gain additional insight into their own biases. Data on disparities should be presented from recent sources or as suggested below. Learners will reflect on their own biases, share as they are able with a partner, and brainstorm as a group how they might be able to limit the impact of such biases.

New in this session: this session introduces two exercises, the IATs and the Imagery exercise, described in Section 5, and two methods, formal presentation and brainstorming, described in Section 4. If these are unfamiliar to you, or you would like tips for usage, you may wish to review the relevant entries.

Session Objectives

After participation in this session, learners should be better able to:
1. define, in contemporary terms, race, ethnicity, and culture (Objective 1 – knowledge)
2. recognize their own potential for bias and stereotyping, be able to identify their own stereotypes and biases (Objective 12 – awareness)
3. explore how their attitudes, biases and stereotypes affect clinical encounters, clinical decision-making and quality of care (Objective 12 – awareness, knowledge)
4. identify and appreciate how clinician bias and stereotyping can affect interactions with patients, families, communities, and other members of the health care team (Objective 13 – awareness)
5. discuss the link between effective communication and quality of care (Objective 13 – awareness, knowledge).

Instructional Materials

Web-based IAT exercise or Sorting People exercise; Imagery exercise (*see* Section 5); data for formal presentation; whiteboard or flip chart for brainstorming; index cards or forms for commitment to change.

Time Schedule

00:00 – 00:05   Session introduction
00:05 – 00:15   Debriefing of computer-based exercises
00:15 – 00:35   Imagery exercise and discussion
00:35 – 00:45   Data review – didactic, examination of data tables, recent article
00:45 – 00:55   Brainstorming
00:55 – 01:00   Session conclusion – commitment to change

Process

1. Introduction (5 minutes): the session introduction serves as an opportunity to introduce presenter and participants if they are not familiar to one another and provides an opportunity to present the session objectives.
2. Debriefing of computer-based exercises (10 minutes): assuming learners completed the IAT prior to the session, this is an opportunity to explore their reactions and any lessons learned about themselves and about stereotyping. We generally use the Gender and Sexual Orientation versions of the IAT, but you should select the ones that resonate with your institution and what is going on locally and nationally. See IAT for instructions in using the exercise. Note: Sorting People from the Public Broadcasting Services (PBS) website[1] can be substituted for the online IAT as an alternative exploration of the limits of our capacity to accurately judge ethnic background based on physical characteristics. *See* Sorting People in Section 5 for instructions on using this exercise.

3. Imagery exercise and discussion (20 minutes): *See* Imagery exercise in Section 5 for details.
4. Data review (10 minutes): the key here is that you select data or reports that relate to your learners. We are supporting the importance of the link between health care providers and health disparities. This should be very brief. There is an abundance of data available, including:
    a) review of an article, e.g. Lauderdale *et al.*[2] or Schulman *et al.*[3]
    b) National Healthcare Disparity Reports[4]
    c) California County Health Status Profiles[5]
    d) results of the first seven years of using the IAT[6]
    e) Institute of Medicine (IOM) Report, Unequal Treatment[7]
5. Brainstorming (10 minutes): the group addresses the question, 'What can health providers do to limit the negative impact of bias and stereotyping on patient care?'
6. Conclusion (5 minutes): conclude with a review of the importance of the session's goals and central learning points, linking these into the results of the brainstorm exercise. Finish with commitment to change where each learner writes at least one thing they will do differently in their care of patients based on what they learned in this session.

Cautionary Note

A key point is that everyone is vulnerable to bias and stereotyping. Learners need not be upset with themselves over this cognitive reality; rather, they should work toward mindful awareness and limiting the impact of bias in clinical encounters and decision-making.

References

1. Public Broadcasting Service. *Sorting People*. Available from: http://www.pbs.org/race/002_SortingPeople/002_00-home.htm
2. Lauderdale DS, Wen M, Jacobs EA, *et al.* Immigrant perceptions of discrimination in health care: the California Health Interview Survey 2003. *Med Care.* 2006 Oct; **44**(10): 914–20.
3. Schulman KA, Berlin JA, Harless W, *et al.* The effect of race and sex on physicians' recommendations for cardiac catheterization. *N Engl J Med.* 1999; **340**: 618–26.
4. Agency for Health Care Quality and Research. *National Healthcare Disparity Reports.* Available from: http://www.ahrq.gov/qual/measurix.htm
5. California Department of Public Health. *County Health Status Profiles.* Available from: http://www.dhs.ca.gov/hisp/chs/OHIR/reports/
6. Results of the first seven years of using the IAT. Available from: http://www.projectimplicit.net/generalinfo.php
7. Smedley BD, Stith AY, Nelson AR, editors. IOM Report: *Unequal Treatment: Confronting Racial and Ethnic Disparities in Health Care.* Board on Health Sciences Policy. Washington, DC: National Academies Press; 2002. Available from: http://www.iom.edu/CMS/3740/4475.aspx

Resources

Gladwell M. *Blink: The power of thinking without thinking.* New York: Little Brown and Company, 2005.
Implicit Association Test (IAT). https://implicit.harvard.edu/implicit/
Project Implicit. http://www.projectimplicit.net/generalinfo.php

SESSION 2 The Culturally Responsive Interview – the BATHE Mnemonic

Session Description

This session is designed to help learners enhance their cultural competence with individual patients and their families. In this session, the BATHE model of the doctor–patient interview is presented (Background, Affect, what Troubles you most, how are you Handling it, and Empathy). A video clip from the American Academy of Family Physicians (AAFP) training video *Quality Care for Diverse Populations* (2002) helps introduce and illustrate how following the BATHE mnemonic facilitates a culturally responsive interview. A brief role play exercise serves to provide hands-on experience with these interviewing skills. At the end of the session, each learner makes a commitment to change that expresses at least one thing they will do differently in their care of patients based on what they learned in this session.

New in this session: this session introduces two teaching methods, use of a video clip and role play, described in more detail in Section 4. Prior to using them, you may wish to review the relevant entries.

Session Objectives

After participation in the session, learners should be better able to:
1. describe at least one model for effective cross-cultural communication and data gathering (Objective 22 – knowledge)
2. describe common challenges in cross-cultural communication (e.g. trust, style) (Objective 22 – knowledge)
3. conduct and document a culturally responsive history within the context of family-centered care, eliciting a cultural, social, and medical history, including a patient's health beliefs and model of their illness (Objective 23 – skill)
4. demonstrate respect for a patient's cultural and health beliefs (Objective 23 – awareness/ attitude).

Instructional Materials

AAFP videotape, *Quality Care for Diverse Populations* (2002) – vignette 1 (the instructional booklet is very useful in understanding how to incorporate their materials into the teaching of interviewing and cultural competence); two role playing scenarios if learners are too junior to have own patients (developed as described in Section 4); forms or index cards for commitment to change.

Time Schedule

00:00 – 00:05   Session introduction
00:05 – 00:15   Didactic presentation: doctor–patient communication
00:15 – 00:30   BATHE video clip and debriefing
00:30 – 00:50   BATHE role play and discussion
00:50 – 00:55   Commitment to change
00:55 – 01:00   Session conclusion

Process

1. Introduction (5 minutes): the session introduction serves as an opportunity to introduce presenter and participants, if they are not familiar to one another. Moreover, it is the opportunity to present the session objectives to the learners, and explain how this session is part of the larger culturally responsive care curriculum.
2. Formal presentation (10 minutes): this brief didactic presentation should focus on the role of respectful, clear communication between doctor and patient in the provision of culturally responsive medical care. Invite the group of learners to collectively offer definitions of 'patient-centered care'. Key points for a presentation might be: a) description of patient-centered care; b) verbal and non-verbal behaviors for connecting with patients; c)

presentation of relevant empirical data; and d) structure of the doctor–patient encounter.

3. Video clip and debriefing (15 minutes): show vignette 1 in AAFP video. Instruct the learners to view the doctor–patient interaction, which exemplifies the implementation of the BATHE mnemonic. At the conclusion, debrief, ask the group a) what did they like most in the physician's style and use of BATHE? and b) what did they see as limitations or problems in the encounter? Here it is helpful to emphasize that mnemonics like BATHE and LEARN (*see* Session 16) serve as a roadmap for navigating the patient encounter. It is incumbent on each learner to experiment with these strategies in the development of their own road map toward effective doctor–patient communication.

4. Role play process (20 minutes): have the BATHE mnemonic (Background, Affect, what Troubles you most, how are you Handling it, and Empathy) written in large letters at the front of the meeting room. Divide learners into pairs, one who will take the role of patient, the other of doctor. Have them move their chairs so that they face each other, but that the learner in the doctor role faces the mnemonic posted at the front. Ask the learner playing the patient to think of a real patient they have worked with, and to be that patient for the exercise (or develop scripts for each 'patient'). Review the following process with the learners. The entire interchange should take approximately five minutes:

    Doctor: begins by welcoming the patient and inquiring as to what brings them in.
    Patient: briefly (in one or two sentences) describes a problem.
    Doctor: inquires more about the problem via the BATHE mnemonic.

    Debrief the exercise by first asking those who played the role of the doctor to comment on what went well in the exercise, and/or what new learning they acquired. Next, ask them to comment on difficulties or challenges. This is followed by feedback from the 'patient' about firstly positive, and then any problematic perceptions of the encounter. This debriefing is most helpful when conducted aloud with the group as a whole, but can be done within the individual pairs. Repeat the role play with a second patient case and debriefing process with the roles reversed. This exercise can be done in triads (doctor, patient, observer) if there is sufficient time for three rounds (three cases required). In this model the large group debriefing is done at the end of the entire exercise.

5. Commitment to change (5 minutes): each learner writes one commitment on an index card (or in a journal if used) that expresses at least one thing they will do differently in their care of patients based on what they learned in this session.

6. Conclusion (5 minutes): conclude with a review of the importance of the session's goals and central learning points, and perhaps with a reading of learners' commitments, inviting learners to take the session contents directly back into their clinical work.

Cautionary Notes

❏ When debriefing the video and/or the role play, insure that both positive and critical impressions (if any) are shared, positive first, and always in a respectful manner aimed toward learning and growth. *See* Section 4 on debriefing and facilitation for details.

❏ Clear guidelines for the role playing exercise will maximize success. *See* Section 4 on role play for details. If you are going to use scripts, keep them short for this exercise, no more than half a page. Include only basic information plus the answers to BATHE.

❏ Occasionally a learner will express an objection to the use of mnemonics – be very open to that sensibility. Mnemonics may not always work, this is just one tool that they might want to try. Acknowledge that their use is often awkward at first, but that once they get integrated into practice they can often be very useful, particularly in a busy clinic or in a difficult encounter.

Resources

Bergeson SC, Dean JD. A systems approach to patient-centered care. *JAMA*. 2006 Dec 20; **296**(23): 2848–51.

Carrillo JE, Green AR, Betancourt JR. Cross-cultural primary care: a patient-based approach. *Ann Intern Med*. 1999 May 18; **130**(10): 829–34.

Levin SJ, Like RC, Gottlieb JC. Useful clinical interviewing mnemonics. *Patient Care*. 2000; **34**: 189–90.

Quality Care for Diverse Populations, video with instructional booklet. Kansas City, MO: American Academy of Family Physicians; 2002.

Stuart MR, Lieberman JA. *The Fifteen Minute Hour: Applied psychotherapy for the primary care physician*. 2nd ed. Westport, CT: Praeger; 1993. (This book first introduced the mnemonic BATHE.)

SESSION 3 Cultural Knowledge – Discussion of a Selected Cultural Group

Session Description

Three sessions (sessions 3, 13, and 23) are designated as annual cultural knowledge sessions. These sessions can be student/resident presentations or faculty presentations. Health professions students and residents do an excellent job in developing these types of sessions. The intent is for the local program to select one cultural group of interest each year, preferably a group that, while present in the greater community, is not part of the clinical practice of the learners. In 2000, 26% of California residents were foreign born. Attached is a data sheet for California and Los Angeles County as a sample, and to provide ideas for ethnic group presentations. At the US census website, Quickfact sheets can be obtained for any state or county and many major cities. In addition to groups selected by country or ethnicity, religious groups could also be the focus for a session, again selected to enlarge the knowledge base of the learners.

New in this session: this session introduces two teaching methods, student/resident presentations and small group activities described in Section 4. If students/residents will be making presentations then the program should consider using the technique of learner portfolios as a means of tracking learner outcomes (*see* portfolio entry in Section 4 for a description).

Session Objectives

After participation in the session, learners should be better able to:
1. value the importance of diversity in health care and address the challenges and opportunities it poses (Objective 3 – attitude)
2. describe historical models of common health beliefs (e.g. illness in the context of 'hot and cold') and identify questions about health practices and beliefs that might be important in a specific local community (Objective 7 – knowledge)
3. discuss race, ethnicity, and culture in the context of the medical interview and health care. Exhibit comfort when conversing with patients/colleagues about cultural issues (Objective 9 – attitude, skill)
4. describe methods to identify key community leaders. Describe strategies for partnering with community activists to eliminate racism and other bias from health care. Collaborate to address community needs (Objective 28 – knowledge, skill).

Instructional Materials

Presentation outline, distributed some weeks prior to the presentation date if learners will be presenting cases, or used to guide the faculty's development of the session; materials requested by learners to facilitate presentations (a list of potential resources is provided); session objectives; small group activity, commitment to change forms or cards.

Time Schedule

00:00 – 00:05 Session introduction
00:05 – 00:20 Presentation of stimulus materials (interview with community member or leader, video clip, panel, quiz/trivia contest, case presentation, etc. *See* entry for Openers in Section 4)
00:20 – 00:40 Formal presentation of information (*see* outline)
00:40 – 00:55 Small group activities: group discussion in relation to a) implications for care of patients; b) community resources; and c) how learners might collaborate with community leaders to address needs
00:55 – 01:00 Session summary and commitment to change

Process

Instructors will want to work with any group of learners in preparing their presentation, particularly if this is their first experience.

1. Session introduction (5 minutes): the instructor can introduce the topic and its place in the overall curriculum and then turn the session over to the students/residents in charge or move directly to the introductory activity.
2. Introductory activity (15 minutes): the initial stimulus material or introductory activity (opener) should engage the audience and introduce the topic and may last from 5 to 15 minutes. Potential methods include: interview with community member or leader, video clip/debriefing, panel, quiz/trivia contest (using teams, audience response system, or paper and pencil), case presentation, etc. In the video resources section (*see* Section 7) there are several sources that provide relevant clips including brief segments from the *Worlds Apart* tapes (Laotian child, African-American man, Mexican-American woman, and Muslim man). Caution: if a video is used it should focus the audience on the objectives for this session.
3. Formal presentation of information (20 minutes): the formal presentation of information can be done using PowerPoint or provided in a handout. PowerPoint allows insertion of a short video clip, photos, quiz items, etc. *See* the attached outline for an overview of the materials to cover if the focus is a cultural group (e.g. African-American, Hispanic), people from a specific country (e.g. Mexico, China); or a specific religious heritage (e.g., Muslim, Buddhist).
4. Small group activities (15 minutes): a minimum of 15 minutes should be scheduled for this activity. Divide the learners into small groups to apply the information provided in the presentation. If the whole group is relatively small, use three groups; assign one item to each group (5–7 minutes). Sample items are: a) implications of the culturally based health beliefs of this group for care of patients; b) community resources for this cultural group; and c) how learners might collaborate with community leaders to address needs. Suggest that the groups agree on three to five points to share. In the follow-up discussion with the entire group, the facilitator should review all three items. Seek input from each of the groups (8–10 minutes).
5. Conclusion and commitment to change (5 minutes): the instructor should thank the learners (if they presented) and request that each person (student/resident presenters and audience) write one commitment and take new insights and knowledge directly back into their clinical work.

Cautionary Note

It is important to emphasize that knowledge learning about other groups helps health care providers develop hypotheses about the cultural background of patients. In the end, providers must strive to hold stereotyping 'at bay' and draw conclusions based on information provided by the patient himself/herself.

SESSION 3 HANDOUT: Cultural Knowledge Presentation Preparation Guidelines

Directions: The portion of the session you lead will be 50 minutes in length. A sample demographic sheet and a resource list are provided for you to use in finding appropriate data and resources. Think of dividing your session into three parts – introductory activity, formal presentation, and small group activity/discussion. Review the description of the session and be sure you understand the session objectives and time schedule.

1. Plan an **introductory activity** (5–15 minutes): the activity should draw the learners toward the topic and make them ready (if not eager) to learn more about the cultural group. Be creative – make it fun for your learners as well as educational. Potential methods include: interview with community member or leader, the exercise 'chicken soup', video clip/ debriefing, panel, quiz/trivia contest (using teams, audience response system, or paper and pencil), case presentation, etc. In the video resources section (Section 7) there are several sources that provide relevant clips including brief segments from the *Worlds Apart* tapes (Laotian child, African-American man, Mexican-American woman, and Muslim man). **Caution**: if a video is used it should focus the audience on the objectives for this session.

2. Plan and rehearse the **formal presentation** (20 minutes). You may want a handout to accompany your PowerPoint to expand on important areas. The PowerPoint should focus on the things most relevant to health beliefs, health disparities, and health care disparities. The talk might be divided into three parts that can be divided equally or with more time spent on the last two sections.

   Overview (6 minutes):
   a) *Country* – language, including number of dialects; any important interpersonal relationship information (e.g. naming, status, roles, greetings, displays of respect, general etiquette); unique information about marriage, family, kinship (marriage, gender roles, extended families); religious beliefs and practices.
   b) *Ethnic Group* – same information as for country with addition of countries of origin.
   c) *Religious Group* – basic tenants in relevant areas of daily living.

   Health beliefs and practices (7 minutes): describe in general or in relation to relevant topics like: a) reproduction (pregnancy, childbirth, post partum practices); b) nutrition and food; c) alcohol, drugs, tobacco; d) attitudes toward death and suffering; e) complementary therapies.

   Disparities and community resources (7 minutes): discuss any data on health disparities in your community, state, or in the nation and provide information about local community leader(s) and community groups/resources serving this community.

3. **Small group activity** (15 minutes): divide the learners into small groups to apply the information provided in the presentation. If the whole group is relatively small, use three groups; assign one item to each group (5–7 minutes). Sample items are: a) implications of the culturally based health beliefs of this group for care of patients; b) community resources for this cultural group; and c) how learners might collaborate with community leaders to address needs. Suggest that the groups agree on three to five points to share. In the follow-up discussion with the entire group the facilitator should address all three items. Seek input from each group (8–10 minutes).

SESSION 3 Sample Ethnic Data Tables – California and Los Angeles

Ethnic Groups in California (2005 Census):
- ❏ Hispanic (35.2%)
- ❏ White Non-Hispanic (43.8%)
- ❏ Asian (12.2%)
- ❏ Black (6.7%)
- ❏ American Indian (1.2%)
- ❏ Native Hawaiian (0.4%)
- ❏ Two or more races (2.4%)

Among Asians in 2000, the Chinese numbered 980,642, or 2.9% of the population. There were also 918,678 Filipinos (2.7%), 447,032 Vietnamese (up from 242,946 in 1990), 345,882 Koreans, 314,819 Asian Indians (up from 112,560), 288,854 Japanese (down from 353,251 in 1990), 55,456 Laotians, 20,571 native Hawaiians (down from 43,418 in 1990), 37,498 Samoans, and 20,918 Guamanians.

Ethnic Groups in Los Angeles (2000 Census):
- ❏ Hispanic (46.5%)
- ❏ White Non-Hispanic (29.7%)
- ❏ Other race (25.7%)
- ❏ Black (11.2%)
- ❏ Two or more races (5.2%)
- ❏ Filipino (2.7%)
- ❏ Korean (2.5%)
- ❏ Chinese (1.7%)
- ❏ American Indian (1.4%)
- ❏ Japanese (1.0%)
- ❏ Other Asian (0.9%)
- ❏ Asian Indian (0.7%)
- ❏ Vietnamese (0.5%)

(Total can be greater than 100% because Hispanics could be counted in other races.)

Source: US Census Data – Quick Facts, State of California, http://quickfacts.census.gov/qfd/states/06000.html

For data on health quality or disparities go to the website of the Agency for Health Care Quality and Research: http://www.ahrq.gov/qual/measurix.htm. Here you will find the annual National Healthcare Disparities Reports (NHDR) and the National Healthcare Quality Report (NHQR). The NHQR addresses the current state of health care quality and the opportunities for improvement for all Americans as a whole, while the NHDR addresses the distribution of improvements in health care quality and access across the different populations that make up the United States.

SESSION 3 Cultural Knowledge Web-Based Resources

A wide variety of health care and educational institutions have websites that provide information about various cultures, religions, and other minority groups. The following websites can be used both for this presentation as well as for enhancing medical care to unfamiliar groups.

http://bearspace.baylor.edu/Charles_Kemp/www/refugees.htm
This site provides resources for cross-cultural care and prevention in relation to a variety of Asian cultures including Burmese, Cambodian/Khmer, Laotian/Lao, Vietnamese, Indian (Asian), as well as information on refugee and immigrant health.

http://www.beliefnet.com/
This site provides useful neutrally written descriptions of 28 different faiths and their belief structures, including Buddhism, Hinduism, Christianity (many variants), Islam, Judaism, Pagan and earth-based Taoism, and Sikhism.

http://www.ethnomed.org/
This site contains culture specific pages as well as pages on cross cultural health topics. The University of Washington maintains the site. The site provides cultural profiles for the following cultural groups: Cambodian, Chinese, Eritrean, Ethiopian (also Oromo and Tigrean people), Hmong, Mexican, Somali, and Vietnamese.

http://www.health.qld.gov.au/multicultural/health_workers/cultdiver_guide.asp
This site provides information about the following cultural groups from the perspective of the health care system in Queensland, Australia: Bosnian Muslims, Cambodians, Chinese, Croatians, Greeks, Hmong, Italians, Muslims from West Asia, Philippines, Samoans, Tongans, Serbians, and Vietnamese.

http://www.healthsystem.virginia.edu/internet/chaplaincy/
This site provides brief helpful descriptions of Buddhism, Hinduism, Islam, Christianity (Protestant, Catholic) and Judaism. It provides a booklet, *Religious Beliefs and Practices Affecting Health Care*, developed for use by UVA Health System staff. Hard copies of the booklet are also available for $3/copy or $30/dozen. The PDF file is also available for $25 and allows the purchaser to make and distribute copies at their own institution.

http://www.hispanichealth.org/
This site has resources for purchase including: *Delivering Health Care to Hispanics: A manual for providers.* 3rd ed. (2004) and the Companion Workbook; and *A Primer for Cultural Proficiency: Towards quality health services for Hispanics* (2001).

http://www.metrokc.gov/health/glbt/
These webpages address the health concerns of gay, lesbian, bisexual, and transgender people, also known as 'GLBT' people and 'sexual minorities'.

Session Description

This session explores the contributors to health and health care disparities. A quiz is used as a warm-up activity. National statistics will be reviewed and extensive discussion will be held in relation to the four contributors as described in the IOM Report, *Unequal Treatment: patient, provider, health care system, and society*.[1] *A Tale of Two Families* from the PBS Race Website[2] will be read to stimulate discussion about historical, political, environmental and societal impacts. Learners will be encouraged to reflect in a journal or commitment to change form on ways each of them can enhance patient encounters to help address their own potential negative or positive impact on disparities.

New in this session: this session introduces two teaching methods, think-write-share (or think-pair-share), and quizzes, games, polls, audience response system (described in Section 4). If these methods are unfamiliar to you, you may wish to review the relevant entries.

Objectives

After participation in the session, learners should be better able to:

1. recognize and describe how access, historical, political, environmental, and institutional factors (including racism and discrimination) impact health and underlie health and health care disparities (Objective 17 – awareness, knowledge)
2. identify how race, ethnicity and social determinants of health (e.g. education, culture, socioeconomic status, housing, and employment) affect health and health care quality, cost, and outcomes (Objective 18 – knowledge)
3. identify and discuss the contributors to disparities (patient, provider, health care system, and society) and discuss the challenges/barriers to eliminating health disparities (Objective 19 – knowledge)
4. describe patterns of health care disparities that can result, at least in part, from clinician bias (Objective 20 – knowledge).

Instructional Materials

Flip chart, pens, tape (unless using Post-a-Note sheets); Quiz and Chart (Death Statistics) from the current *Health, United States Report* (attached handout is from the 2007 document).[3]

Time Schedule

00:00 – 00:05 Warm-up activity – quiz
00:05 – 00:20 Review actual data, think-write-share, overview of session objectives
00:20 – 00:40 Small group (four contributors – patient, provider, health care system, and society – one area per group) and debriefing
00:40 – 00:55 Read *A Tale of Two Families*,[2] and facilitation of general discussion
00:55 – 01:00 Conclusion and commitment to change

Process

1. Quiz (5 minutes): the session begins with a quiz on health care disparities (attached). The learners complete the quiz and depending on program purpose they can be collected with names or kept by learners.
2. Objectives and think-write-share (15 minutes): quickly review the objectives for the session. Have each learner find a partner. Distribute a color-coded answer sheet for the quiz (attached); a selected section from the US annual *National Healthcare Disparities Report* (select one that is meaningful for your community – we suggest the tables on heart disease, pages 45–49 or the quality summary tables, pages 85–89 of the 2006 edition);[4] and several questions to answer. Have them think and write together. Leave a couple of minutes at the end to share answers. Capture the learners' impressions of the data. Sample questions:
   a) What do you learn by looking at the death statistics provided in the 2006 *Health, United*

States Report[3] about the relative status of varying racial/ethnic groups? Which group is doing the best? Which is the worst?

b) What are the four leading causes of death among Hispanics?

c) In looking at the section from the *2006 National Healthcare Disparities Report*,[4] are disparities for Hispanics generally decreasing or increasing in the area of quality (or heart disease)?

d) List three questions that are raised in your mind as you look at these data in regard to health and health care disparities?

3. Small groups and debriefing (20 minutes): divide the learners into four groups. Each group can gather around a large piece of poster paper attached to the wall. Assign each group one of the four contributors to health and health care disparities: patient, provider, health care system, and society. Ask each group to write down as many factors as they can think of in their assigned area (about 5 minutes). Debrief the activity by having each group present, with other groups adding their input (10–12 minutes). You may want to provide a handout with a sample listing based on the IOM Report, Unequal Treatment and note any additional factors overlooked by the groups (3–5 minutes).

4. *A Tale of Two Families* (15 minutes): read aloud the *Tale of Two Families*[2] – be sure to read the subtitles between sections. It is very effective to have two readers throughout – each speaking in one of the two voices with the instructor announcing each subtitle. Facilitate a brief discussion on the social determinants of health (e.g. education, culture, socioeconomic status, housing, and employment) and how they might affect health and health care quality.

5. Conclusion and commitment to change (5 minutes): this provides learners with an opportunity to reflect and write one thing they will do differently in their clinical practice to minimize their contribution to health disparities. Summarize take-home points.

References

1. Smedley BD, Stith AY, Nelson AR, editors. *Unequal Treatment: Confronting Racial and Ethnic Disparities in Health Care.* Board on Health Sciences Policy. Washington, DC: National Academies Press; 2002. Available from: http://www.iom.edu/CMS/3740/4475.aspx

2. PBS. *Where Race Lives* page – website: http://www.pbs.org/race/000_About/002_06_b-godeeper.htm By clicking on 'A Tale of Two Families' you will explore 'where race lives' by looking at two individuals and how their 'race' affected their family wealth.

3. 2007 *Health, United States Report with Chartbook on Trends in the Health of Americans.* Available from the website of the US Centers for Disease Control: www.cdc.gov/nchs/data/hus/hus07.pdf

4. 2006 *National Healthcare Disparities Report (NHDR).* Available from the website of the US Agency for Health Care Quality and Research: http://www.ahrq.gov/qual/measurix.htm

Resources

Kilbourne AM, Switzer G, Hyman K, *et al.* Advancing health disparities research within the health care system: a conceptual framework. *Am J Public Health.* 2006 Dec; **96**(12): 2113–21.

SESSION 4 Quiz – Relative Mortality by Race/Ethnicity

Directions: For each health indicator, please mark an **H** for the group with the highest level of mortality and an **L** for the group with the lowest level of mortality.

TABLE 3.1 Mortality Rates – Age Adjusted per 100 000 Population by Leading Cause, Year, and Race or Ethnicity, US

Indicator and Year	White Non-Hispanic	Black or African-American	Hispanic or Latino	Am. Indian or Alaska Native	Asian/Pacific Islander
Death rates – all causes, 2004					
Disease of the heart, 2004					
Ischemic heart disease, 2004					
Cerebrovascular disease, 2004					
Malignant neoplasm, 2004					
Trachea, bronchus, lung cancer, 2004					
Colon, rectum and anus cancer, 2004					
Prostate cancer (male), 2004					
Breast cancer (female), 2004					
Chronic lower respiratory diseases, 2004					
Influenza and pneumonia, 2004					
Chronic liver disease and cirrhosis, 2004					
Diabetes mellitus, 2004					
HIV/AIDS, 2004					
Unintentional injuries, 2004					
Motor vehicle injuries, 2004					
Suicide, 2004					
Homicide, 2004					

Source: Table 29 from *Health, United States Report 2007 with Chartbook on Trends in the Health of Americans.* Available from the website of the US Centers for Disease Control: www.cdc.gov/nchs/data/hus/hus07.pdf

Quiz – Answer Sheet for Relative Mortality by Race/ Ethnicity

TABLE 3.2 Mortality Rates – Age Adjusted per 100 000 Population by Leading Cause, Year, and Race or Ethnicity, US

Indicator and Year	White Non-Hispanic	Black or African-American	Hispanic or Latino	Am. Indian or Alaska Native	Asian/Pacific Islander
Death rates – all causes, 2004	786.3	1027.3	586.7	685	443.9
Disease of the heart, 2004	213.3	280.6	158.4	160.2	117.8
Ischemic heart disease, 2004	149.2	179.8	119.2	114.1	84.1
Cerebrovascular disease, 2004	48	69.9	38.2	34.6	41.3
Malignant neoplasm 2004	184.4	227.2	121.9	119.3	110.5
Trachea, bronchus, lung cancer, 2004	53.6	59.8	22.4	31.3	26.2
Colon, rectum and anus cancer, 2004	17.6	24.7	12.6	11.8	11.3
Prostate cancer (male), 2004	23.4	55.5	19.1	17.8	11.4
Breast cancer (female), 2004	23.9	32.2	15.6	14	12.7
Chronic lower respiratory diseases, 2004	43.2	28.2	18.4	31.7	14.7
Influenza and pneumonia, 2004	19.6	22.3	17.1	24.1	16
Chronic liver disease and cirrhosis, 2004	9.2	7.9	14	22.6	3.2
Diabetes mellitus, 2004	22.3	48	32.1	43.7	16.6
HIV/AIDS, 2004	2.3	20.4	5.2	2.5	0.7
Unintentional injuries, 2004	38.8	36.3	29.8	56.4	16.7
Motor vehicle injuries, 2004	15.6	14.8	14.4	28.1	7.8
Suicide, 2004	12	5.3	5.9	10	5.8
Homicide, 2004	3.6	20.1	7.2	7.3	2.5

*Group with highest mortality highlighted in light grey, with the lowest highlighted in dark grey.

Source: Table 29 from *Health, United States Report 2007 with Chartbook on Trends in the Health of Americans*. Available from the website of the US Centers for Disease Control: www.cdc.gov/nchs/data/hus/hus07.pdf

SESSION 4 Reference Sheet for Instructors: Contributors to Health Care Disparities

Patient Factors
- ❏ Genetics
- ❏ Risk behaviors/healthy behaviors
- ❏ Health literacy
- ❏ Treatment refusal
- ❏ Patient preferences/health beliefs
- ❏ Family/social support/spirituality
- ❏ Health seeking (personality, education, income, etc.)

Provider Factors
- ❏ Bias and stereotypes
- ❏ Beliefs about behavior or health of patient
- ❏ Reaction to time pressure
- ❏ Clinical uncertainty
- ❏ Cultural competence (BATHE, LEARN)
- ❏ Language/skill in working with interpreters
- ❏ General medical knowledge and skill
- ❏ Skill in reflection and Practice-Based Learning and Improvement (PBLI)

Health Care System Factors
- ❏ Access/availability and mix of providers
- ❏ Interpretation/translation services provided
- ❏ Profit motive/altruistic motive
- ❏ Time pressures on providers
- ❏ In-service training (providers and staff)
- ❏ Institutional culture
- ❏ Capacity for reflection and continuous quality improvement
- ❏ Fragmentation of financing and delivery

Society Factors
- ❏ Poverty/wealth
- ❏ Racism and other societal prejudices
- ❏ Insurance/sources of payment
- ❏ Resource distribution within health care (geographic, socioeconomic, age, sex)
- ❏ Citizen safety (accidents, homicides, suicides)
- ❏ Community

Source: Smedley BD, Stith AY, Nelson AR, editors. *Unequal Treatment: Confronting Racial and Ethnic Disparities in Health Care (IOM Report).* Board on Health Sciences Policy. Washington, DC: National Academies Press; 2002. Available from: http://www.iom.edu/CMS/3740/4475. aspx

SESSION 5 Disparities Related to Sexual Orientation

Session Description

This session consists of a conversation with GLBTQ (gay, lesbian, bisexual, transgender, queer) individuals and family members who can share their experiences in relation to health care. Data is also provided in relation to special health issues of the GLBTQ population as well as known health and health care disparities. Learners are encouraged to reflect on ways each of them can enhance their interactions with and improve care provided to GLBTQ patients.

New in this session: this session introduces the teaching method, facilitation described in Section 4. If it is unfamiliar to you, you may wish to review the relevant entry.

Session Objectives

After participation in this session, learners should be better able to:

1. recognize and describe how access, historical, political, environmental and institutional factors (including homophobia, heterosexism, and discrimination) impact health and underlie health and health care disparities (Objective 17 – awareness, knowledge)
2. identify and discuss key areas of disparities described in *Healthy People 2010*[1] and the IOM Report,[2] and discuss barriers to eliminating health disparities (Objective 18 – knowledge)
3. describe patterns of health care disparities that can result, at least in part, from clinician bias, recognize disparities that are amenable to intervention and value eliminating disparities (Objective 20 – awareness, knowledge)
4. describe systemic and medical-encounter issues related to health care disparities, including communication issues, clinical decision-making, and patient preferences (Objective 21 – knowledge).

Instructional Materials

Presenters who are GLBTQ, or who have family members who are, and have experience facilitating group discussions on these issues. In Los Angeles, staff members from Gays and Lesbians Initiating Dialogue for Equality (GLIDE) conduct the presentation (contact information: (310) 358-5165, http://www.socal-glide.org); two flip charts and markers (or electronic equivalent). A national resource is Parents, Families and Friends of Lesbians and Gays (PFLAG), http://www.pflag.org.

Time Schedule

00:00 – 00:05   Session introduction
00:05 – 00:25   Facilitation of GLBTQ stereotype exercise
00:25 – 00:50   Panel presentation and discussion
00:50 – 00:55   Commitment to change
00:55 – 01:00   Session conclusion

Process

1. Introduction (5 minutes): the session introduction serves as an opportunity to introduce any guest presenters to the participants.
2. Facilitation of GLBTQ stereotype exercise (20 minutes): the objective of this exercise is to debunk myths the learners may have about GLBTQ communities. The skilled facilitator begins by soliciting beliefs the learners may have about origins of homosexuality, typical professions held by gay men and lesbians, sexuality and sexual practices and relationships. In response to these, data is presented to provide a realistic, data-based portrayal of these communities. To prompt group discussion (which is often particularly difficult in this area), facilitators may ask questions such as:
   - what other terms are used to describe persons who identify as GLBTQ, including derogatory terms?
   - what is known about the origins of sexual identity and lifestyles?
   - what types of sexual behavior do GLBT persons engage in?
   - where do gay and lesbian people live?

- what types of jobs do they have?
- how do all of these aspects compare to those of heterosexual orientation?
3. Panel presentation and discussion (25 minutes): this is an opportunity for learners to interact with gay and lesbian individuals and their family members. Panelists are invited to share experiences (both positive and negative) with the health care system. For example, gay and lesbian partners are often not recognized as family members of ill, hospitalized patients. Panelists are encouraged to describe 'optimal' doctor–patient encounters that exemplify culturally sensitive care, and learners are encouraged to ask questions and engage in dialogue.
4. Commitment to change (5 minutes): each learner writes one commitment on a form, index card (or in a journal if used) that expresses one thing the person will do differently to enhance their care of GLBTQ patients, based on what they learned in this session.
5. Session conclusion (5 minutes): conclude with a review of the importance of the session's goals and central learning points, and perhaps with a reading of learners' commitments, inviting learners to take the session contents directly back into their clinical work.

Cautionary Notes

❏ This topic can be quite uncomfortable for learners. The discussion facilitation must be done by someone with training and experience (e.g. *see* GLIDE website).

❏ Panelists must be coached to speak directly to issues associated with the objectives of the session.

❏ It can be valuable to have a discussion about how a health care professional goes about providing excellent care to a gay or lesbian patient while holding strong religious beliefs that do not condone homosexuality.

❏ Do not assume that all audience members are heterosexual.

References

1. *Healthy People 2010*. Available from: http://www.healthypeople.gov/Document/tableofcontents.htm
2. Smedley BD, Stith AY, Nelson AR, editors. *Unequal Treatment: Confronting Racial and Ethnic Disparities in Health Care*. Board on Health Sciences Policy. Washington, DC: National Academies Press; 2002. Available from: http://www.iom.edu/CMS/3740/4475.aspx

Resources

Bakker LJ, Cavender A. Promoting culturally competent care for gay youth. *J School Nurs*. 2003 Apr; 19(2): 65–72.

Crisp C. The gay affirmative practice scale (GAP): a new measure for assessing cultural competence with gay and lesbian clients. *Soc Work*. 2006 Apr; 51(2): 115–26.

Kaiser Permanente. *A Provider's Handbook on Culturally Competent Care: Lesbian, gay, bisexual and transgender population*. Los Angeles, CA: Kaiser Permanente; 2000.

McGarry K, Clarke J, Cyr MG. Enhancing residents' cultural competence through a lesbian and gay health curriculum. *Acad Med*. 2000 May; 75(5): 515.

Meyer I, Northridge M. *The Health of Sexual Minorities: Public health perspectives on lesbian, gay, bisexual and transgender populations*. New York: Springer Publications; 2006.

SESSION 6 Building Cultural Skills: Complementary/ Alternative Care, the ETHNIC Mnemonic

Session Description

This skill-building session introduces the interviewing mnemonic ETHNIC (Explanation, Treatment, Healers [traditional], Negotiate, Intervention, Collaboration). The session opens with segment four of the American Academy of Family Physicians video, *Quality Care for Diverse Populations*, which introduces the mnemonic. This is followed by a progressive interview with a standardized patient (SP), to provide residents with group practice using the mnemonic. The learners will then practice individually through a role play exercise. At the end of the session a handout that provides information about health beliefs common to various immigrant populations will be distributed to extend learners' cultural knowledge.

New in this session: this session introduces the teaching method, 'use of standardized patients' described in Section 4. If this technique is unfamiliar to you, you should review the relevant entry.

Session Objectives

After participation in the session, learners should be better able to:
1. identify questions about health practices and beliefs that might be important in a specific local community (Objective 7 – knowledge)
2. identify healing traditions and beliefs of patients and/or their families, including ethno-medical beliefs (Objective 8 – skill)
3. ask questions in a non-judgmental manner to elicit patient preferences, listen and respond appropriately to patient feedback about key cross-cultural issues (Objective 8 – attitude, skill)
4. elicit information about ethno-medical conditions and ethno-medical healers (Objective 8 – skill)
5. assess and enhance patient adherence based on the patient's explanatory model. Describe ways to enhance patient adherence by collaborating with traditional/community healers (Objective 25 – knowledge, skill).

Instructional Materials

Quality Care for Diverse Populations video, segment four (ETHNIC); VCR and projection system; SP case and trained patient; photocopies of two role playing scenarios; handout on health beliefs.

Time Schedule

00:00 – 00:05   Session introduction
00:05 – 00:20   Video: the ETHNIC mnemonic and debriefing
00:20 – 00:40   Progressive interview with an SP
00:40 – 00:55   Role play using the ETHNIC mnemonic
00:55 – 01:00   Commitment to change and session conclusion

Process

An appropriate SP case should be selected prior to the session or develop an SP case appropriate for use with the ETHNIC mnemonic. Train the SP to be able to answer all questions that might be asked within the context of using ETHNIC. Try to select a case where a traditional healer was used. If you do not have the resources to hire an SP, then the instructor or senior resident can be trained to play the role.
1. Introduction (5 minutes): Introduce this session with a story from personal experience of a challenge in your own family when family health beliefs conflicted with recommended life style changes or recommended care, or use a challenge with one of your prior patients.
2. Video presentation and discussion (15 minutes): this brief didactic presentation focuses on the importance of understanding a patient's world view when assessing a problem and in

formulating a treatment plan. The ETHNIC mnemonic is presented to the learners in the video. In a brief group brainstorming exercise, solicit examples of various group health beliefs and healing traditions.

3. Skills practice – progressive interview with a SP (20 minutes): the progressive interview uses a time-in/time-out technique to control the instruction as the learners take turns as the interviewer.

   a) Rules need to be established in terms of who can call a 'time-out'. Generally, only the current 'interviewer' or the instructor can call a time-out (by making a 'T' with his/her two hands). During a time-out, the SP bows his/her head and is 'not in the room'. When time-in is called, the patient returns to the point in the interview where the time-out was called with no apparent interruption to the interview.

   b) Once the interview begins, the current interviewer can call time out to ask for advice from the other students. The instructor can call time out to make a point or to change interviewer.

   c) The interview generally moves fairly quickly, no more than a couple of minutes per learner.

   d) After each learner (or about five learners if the group is large) has had an opportunity to interview the SP, the instructor leads a discussion of the process and the main learning points. Learners may provide feedback to each other as time permits.

4. Role play (15 minutes): have the ETHNIC mnemonic written in large letters at the front of the classroom (see Figure 3.1). Divide learners into pairs, one who will take the role of patient, the other of doctor. Have them move their chairs so that they face each other, such that the learner in the doctor role faces the mnemonic posted at the front.

   a) Ask the learner playing the patient to think of a real patient they have worked with, and to be that patient for the exercise (or develop your own case or use the case provided). Review the following process with the learners. The entire interchange should take approximately 5 minutes:

   Doctor: begins by welcoming the patient and inquiring as to what brings them in.
   Patient: briefly (one or two sentences) describes the problem.
   Doctor: works through the problem with the patient using the ETHNIC mnemonic.

   b) Each team switches roles and completes the second role play.

   c) Debrief – first ask those who played the role of the doctor to comment on what went well in the exercise, and/or what new learning they acquired. Next, ask them to comment on difficulties or challenges. This is followed by feedback from the 'patient' about positive (first) and then any problematic perceptions of the encounter. Learners can be challenged to begin to consider how they might negotiate a treatment plan incorporating both patient health beliefs and their medical knowledge. This debriefing is most helpful when conducted aloud with the group as a whole, but can be done within the individual pairs. This exercise can be done in triads (doctor, patient, observer) if there is sufficient time for three rounds (three cases required). In this model the large group debriefing is done at the end of the entire exercise.

5. Commitment to change and conclusion (5 minutes): each learner writes at least one thing they will do differently in their care of patients based on what they learned in this session. Conclude with a review of the central learning points, and invite learners to take the session contents directly back into their clinical work. Here it is helpful to emphasize that mnemonics like BATHE and ETHNIC serve as a roadmap for navigating the patient encounter. It is incumbent on each learner to experiment with these strategies in the development of their own roadmap toward effective doctor–patient communication.

Cautionary Notes
❏ When debriefing the video and/or the role play, insure that both positive and critical impressions (if any) are shared, positive first, and always in a respectful manner aimed toward learning and growth. See debriefing entry in Section 4 for details.
❏ Clear guidelines for the role playing exercise will maximize success. See role play entry in Section 4 for details.
❏ Occasionally a learner will express an objection to the use of mnemonics – be very open to that sensibility. Acknowledge that their use is often awkward at first, but that once they

get integrated into practice they can often be very useful, particularly in a busy clinic or in a difficult encounter.

References

1. http://www.watchtower.org
2. http://adam.about.com/care/Jehovahs-Witnesses-position-overview.htm?once=true&

Resources

Kobylarz FA, Heath JM, Like RC. The ETHNIC(S) mnemonic: a clinical tool for ethnogeriatric education. *J Am Geriatr Soc*. 2002 Sep; **50**(9): 1582–9.

Levin SJ, Like RC, Gottlieb JC. Useful clinical interviewing mnemonics. *Patient Care*. 2000; **34**: 189–90.

Like RC. Culturally competent family medicine: transforming clinical practice and ourselves. *Am Fam Physician*. 2005 Dec; **72**(11): 2189.

Quality Care for Diverse Populations, video with instruction booklet. Kansas City, MO: American Academy of Family Physicians; 2002. (Training manual very useful in understanding how to incorporate the materials into teaching interviewing and cultural competence.)

E	Explanation (how do you explain your illness?)
T	Treatment (what treatment have you tried?)
H	Healers (have you sought any advice from complementary or alternative medicine providers/healers?)
N	Negotiate (mutually acceptable options)
I	Intervention (agree on)
C	Collaboration (with patient, family, and healers)

FIGURE 3.1 The ETHNIC Model (Like, 2000) The ETHNIC mnemonic is an example of a simple framework for practicing culturally competent care.

Role Play Cases

Case 1

Doctor: Your patient has a very low blood count, and you are considering admission to the hospital for transfusion.

Patient: You have a very low blood count, and the doctor is considering admitting you to the hospital for transfusion. To begin the session, you present two cards to your doctor (*see* Figure 3.2 and Figure 3.3).

NO BLOOD TRANSFUSION!

As a God-fearing Christian and a believer of Jehovah's word, the Bible, I hereby demand that blood, in any way, shape or form is NOT to be fed into my body; however, blood substitutes may be used in case of extreme loss of blood.

'You must not eat the blood of any sort of flesh'

Leviticus 17:14 NW

Signature:..

Witness:.. (Over)

FIGURE 3.2 'No blood transfusion!' card.[1]

Jehovah's Witnesses' basic position on blood

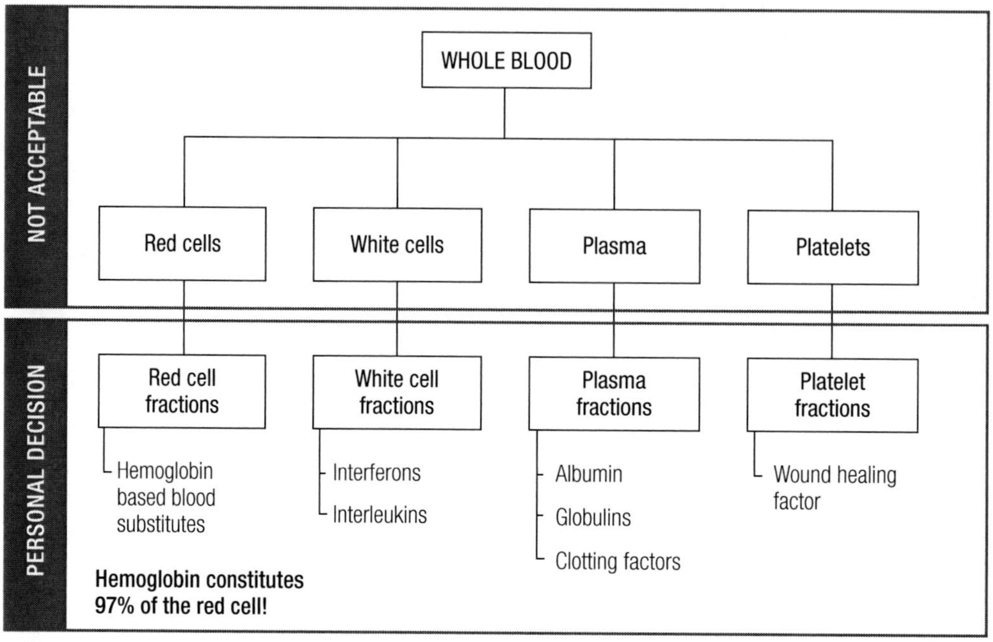

FIGURE 3.3 Jehovah's Witnesses' Basic Position on Blood.[2]

Case 2

Doctor: Your patient has very painful arthritis and you are considering pain medications.
Patient: Your grandmother was a Yaqui Indian healer. You are not interested in taking any medications, yet your arthritis is very painful. You prefer prayer and herbal approaches.

SESSION 7 Precepting Self and Others: Using the Cultural Competency SOAP Grid

Session Description

The focus of this session is on encouraging the learners to precept themselves and each other in relation to cultural competency through use of a tool, the Cultural Competence (CC) SOAP Grid. The CC SOAP Grid (attached) was designed to offer a number of 'onramps' to discussion of cultural issues in a typical patient case. The body of the grid is comprised of specific questions for the resident/student regarding the **Subjective, Objective, Assessment**, and **Plan** components of a case. There is also an additional row entitled **Post-Hoc Reflection** that provides a number of 'big picture' follow-up questions about culture and patient care.

For the horizontal axis of the grid, we selected three thematic areas which merit attention in caring for culturally diverse patients: 1) the degree to which this case reflects or might become an instance of a **Health Disparity** or inequitable care; 2) the degree to which **Medical Errors** are possible and can be prevented in the provision of care to this patient; and 3) the degree to which the intervention is reflective of a **Patient-Centered Care** model of doctoring. We want to encourage learners to take the classroom activities out into their clinical settings and the CC SOAP Grid is one tool to encourage that purpose.

New in this session: this session introduces one tool, the CC SOAP Grid. If this is unfamiliar to you, you may wish to review the relevant entry in Section 6.

Session Objectives

After participation in the session, learners should be better able to:
1. discuss race, ethnicity, and culture in the context of the medical interview and health care (Objective 9 – awareness, knowledge)
2. exhibit comfort when conversing with colleagues about cultural issues (Objective 9 – skill)
3. value the importance of curiosity, empathy, and respect in patient care (Objective 11 – attitude)
4. describe the underlying factors and the impact of race/ethnicity, culture, and class on clinical decision-making (Objective 14 – knowledge).

Instructional Materials

Alicia Mercado tape from the *Worlds Apart* Video Series (*see* Video Resources in Section 7); projection equipment; flip chart (large Post-a-Note pad often works best) and pens; blank sheets of paper; a copy of the CC SOAP Grid for each learner. Prior to the start of the session, tape four sheets of flip chart paper to the wall, labeling them S, O, A, and P. If your group has more than 10–12 learners, put up two sheets for each letter.

Time Schedule

00:00 – 00:05 Session introduction
00:05 – 00:20 Video clip and discussion
00:20 – 00:30 Silent exercise – brainstorming
00:30 – 00:50 Debriefing and introduction to the CC SOAP Grid
00:50 – 00:55 Commitment to change

Process

1. Introduction (5 minutes): the session introduction serves as an opportunity to introduce presenter and participants and present the session objectives. As a warm-up you may want to remind the learners about the mnemonic BATHE (Background, Affect, what Troubles you most, How are you handling it, and Empathy) from Session 2.
2. Video clip and discussion (5 minutes): provide a blank sheet of paper to each learner and direct them to write the letters SOAP down the left-hand side (spacing them so there will be room for notes). Ask them to watch the patient encounter in the video clip and

write whatever they learn in relation to the Subjective, Objective, Assessment and Plan components beside the appropriate letter. View the first 5 minutes only of the *Worlds Apart* video, the Alicia Mercado story (the initial doctor–patient encounter only, *see* Video Resources in Section 7).

Discussion (10 minutes): walk over to the 'S' sheet posted on the wall and ask for anything the learners know about the patient. Write the answers in small print near the top. Do the same for the O, A, and P. Acknowledge that we don't know enough. Explain that we are going to provide them with a tool that they can use to precept themselves to encourage their own growth in relation to providing patient-centered culturally competent care, avoiding medical errors and hopefully helping to address health care disparities. However, before we do that we want them to think about Alicia Mercado and the questions that they have about her.

3. Silent brainstorming exercise (10 minutes): instructions to students: 'We have just been assigned to Mrs Mercado's care team. In preparation for talking with her, we are preparing a list of the questions that need to be answered in order to care for her. We have arbitrarily decided that these questions should go under the SOAP rubric'. Hand out marking pens and ask learners to silently move to one of the posted sheets. They will need to take turns writing. Instruct the group to write the questions about Alicia that need to be answered in order to provide excellent care. Each question should only be listed once. Tell them that they have 10 minutes. Each person should sit down once all his/her questions have been posted (by anyone) on the various sheets around the room.

4. Debriefing and introduction to CC SOAP Grid (20 minutes): Hand out the CC SOAP Grid and select one section to review. Alternately review the questions they have posted with the ones on the grid. Encourage the learners to make up their own CC SOAP Grid or to use the one provided to precept themselves and each other as they work with culturally diverse patients. As they look at the two lists, ask them to put themselves in the place of the provider in the film. If the provider asked herself these questions, how might it impact care?

5. Commitment to change (5 minutes): each learner writes a statement that expresses at least one thing they will do differently in their care of patients based on what they learned in this session.

Instructor Note

Given the complicated nature of the SOAP grid, this session's debriefing requires a skilled facilitator. Less experienced facilitators may wish to read the section on facilitation in Section 4.

Resources
Disparities

Betancourt JR, Maina AW. The Institute of Medicine report 'Unequal Treatment': implications for academic health centers. *Mt Sinai J Med*. 2004 Oct; **71**(5): 314–21.

Horner RD, Salazar W, Geiger HJ, *et al*. Working Group on Changing Health Care Professionals' Behavior. Changing healthcare professionals' behaviors to eliminate disparities in healthcare: What do we know? How might we proceed? *Am J Manag Care*. 2004 Sep; **10** Spec No: SP12–9.

Taylor SL, Lurie N. The role of culturally competent communication in reducing ethnic and racial healthcare disparities. *Am J Manag Care*. 2004 Sep; **10** Spec No: SP1–4.

Medical Errors

Flores G, Ngui E. Racial/ethnic disparities and patient safety. *Pediatr Clin North Am*. 2006 Dec; **53**(6): 1197–215.

Institute of Medicine Report: *To Err is Human: Building A Safer Health System*. Linda Kohn, Janet M. Corrigan, Molla S. Donaldson (editors) Committee on Quality of Care in America, National Academy Press, 1999.

Patient-Centered Care

Betancourt JR. Cultural competence and medical education: many names, many perspectives, one goal. *Acad Med*. 2006 Jun; **81**(6): 499–501.

Carrillo JE, Green AR, Betancourt JR. Cross-cultural primary care: a patient-based approach. *Ann Intern Med*. 1999 May 18; **130**(10): 829–34.

Larson L. Is your hospital culturally competent? (And what does that mean exactly?) *Trustee*. 2005 Feb; **58**(2): 20–3.

Cultural Competence SOAP Grid Handout

The CC SOAP Grid was designed to offer a number of 'onramps' to discussion of cultural issues in a typical patient case. The body of the grid is comprised of specific questions for the resident/student regarding the Subjective, Objective, Assessment, and Plan components of a case. There is also an additional row entitled Post-Hoc Reflection that provides a number of 'big picture' follow-up questions about culture and patient care. The columns of the grid include three thematic areas that merit attention in caring for culturally diverse patients: 1) the degree to which this case reflects or might become an instance of a health disparity or inequitable care; 2) the degree to which medical errors are possible and can be prevented in the provision of care to this patient; and 3) the degree to which the intervention is reflective of a patient-centered care model of doctoring. We encourage learners to use the CC SOAP Grid as one tool to precept themselves.

	Health Disparities	Medical Errors	Patient-Centered Care
Subjective	Did patient self-identify gender, race, age, ethnicity, marital status, sexual orientation, etc? If not, how did you determine the patient's demographics? Considering evidence-based medical literature, is the patient empirically at risk for any health disparities?	Any missing data due to assumptions made? Think about your life context in comparison to that of the patient. Any blind spots? Did you encounter any language issues? How did you handle them? Did patient appear distrustful of the health care system? Were you able to establish a relationship of trust with the patient? If not, what next?	Did you ask about the patient's health beliefs? (Q2: 'What do you think made you sick?' and 'What do you think could help you get better?') What parts of the patient's story require follow up in the next visit?
Objective	Do your exam and lab data address all of the patient's disparity risks (e.g. BMI for overweight patients)?	Did you defer, delay or eliminate any aspect of the physical exam for reasons of your discomfort or patient refusal (e.g. for cultural, religious, gender preferences)? What should your next step be?	Did you feel uncomfortable at any time while conducting physical exam? How did it impact the exam? What should you do to grow from this experience? Did the patient appear uncomfortable during your exam? If so, how did you address the patient's feelings?
Assessment	How does your assessment address cultural differences in disease manifestation? How have you considered any 'problems behind the current medical issue' related to the patient's life context (e.g. homelessness, abuse, poverty, family, substance use)?	Have you made any untested assumptions about this patient that will influence your differential diagnosis or final assessment?	In your assessment/ problem list, do you address the patient's reasons for coming to the clinic? Does the patient understand and agree with your assessment, and how do you know? Are there any discrepancies between your assessment and the patient's health belief system? Describe.
Plan	How have you used knowledge of health disparities in creating your plan? How did you insure that the patient is able and willing to adhere to the plan, within his/her life context?	Is anything omitted from your plan based on 'who' this patient is (e.g. likeable, deserving, etc)? Did you encounter any literacy or language issues? How did you handle them?	Any concerns about the patient's ability or willingness to adhere to the treatment plan, and how did you negotiate issues with the patient? How did you address any patient concerns regarding potential adverse effects of your treatment plan?
Post-Hoc Reflection	Was there a health care disparity already affecting the patient's health status prior to the patient visit?	What are the special communication needs of our patient? Do any require follow-up with other health care providers?	What is your plan to become more knowledgeable and skillful in regard to this patient's special population?

cont.

	Health Disparities	Medical Errors	Patient-Centered Care
Post-Hoc Reflection (*cont.*)	How did the assessment and plan change based on the discussion of health disparities? How can we avoid health disparities for future patients?	Are we at risk for poor outcomes based on patient's health practices (e.g. complementary and alternative medication)?	What went well and what did not work in your negotiation with this patient? How can models with acronyms like ETHNIC and LEARN assist you in your care of patients?

The CC SOAP Grid can also be used to enhance outpatient precepting. It provides questions that the preceptor can ask the student or resident. Students and residents are encouraged to present cases and seek help with cultural and interpersonal challenges in the same way they seek guidance for challenging diagnostic or treatment situations.

SESSION 8 Focused Review of Local, State, and National Health Data (Accidents, Homicide, and Suicide)

Session Description

This annual session (sessions 8, 18 and 28) is designed to provide the opportunity for learners to review actual health status data, national, state, and particularly local. In the state of California, data is provided annually that compare each county with all other counties, with the state average, and with the *Healthy People 2010* goal for a variety of health issues. This data should be reviewed (check you own state Department of Health for similar data) along with any data collected in relation to PBLI (practice-based learning and improvement) goals for your program's clinic or hospital. Learners may also be able to look at the data on their own patient population in relation to program goals or *Healthy People 2010* goals. *Healthy People 2010* is a very extensive document addressing a wide variety of issues. Familiarity with both it and the *Healthy People Midcourse Review* will increase understanding of the goals and of the progress from 2000 to 2005. Since this is an annual session, the program has the opportunity to select different areas of emphasis each year, providing a variety of foci for learner review.

New in this session: this session introduces the teaching technique of 'openers'.

Session Objectives

After participation in the session, learners should be better able to:
1. identify patterns of national data on health, health care disparities, and quality of health care, and describe them in a worldwide immigration context (Objective 4 – knowledge)
2. discuss the epidemiology of health and health care disparities for the local community using *Healthy People 2010* and other resources (Objective 5 – knowledge, skill)
3. critically appraise the literature as it relates to health disparities, including systems issues and quality in health care (Objective 26 – skill).

Instructional Materials

National, regional, and *Healthy People 2010* data (copies made for each person or each small group); local hospital, clinic, and individual resident data if available; small group assignments for this session based on the data focus selected.

Time Schedule

00:00 – 00:05   Session introduction
00:05 – 00:30   Small group data review
00:30 – 00:50   Facilitation of group discussion on common themes
00:50 – 01:00   Conclusion of session, journal or commitment to change

Process

Prior to Session

   a) Select the topic for data review from those included in *Healthy People 2010*. Select a topic that resonates with the local community. Attached are several suggestions.
   b) Plan a relevant small group assignment that requires the students/residents to review the data in a meaningful manner (sample assignment attached).
1. Introduction (5 minutes): this session should begin with an opener that draws the learners' attention to the focus of the session. A quote or a statistic could open the session, or the learners could be presented with a challenge in relation to health care within the clinic, health center or community where data would be important in addressing an issue.
2. Small group exercises – data review (25 minutes): provide the pre-planned assignment to each group along with the data sheets prepared in advance. Monitor the progress of the groups and provide assistance in examining the data if required.
3. Debriefing of exercise and discussion of common themes/challenges (20 minutes): use

facilitation to debrief the exercise. Be careful to include all groups in reporting the answers to the questions in your pre-planned exercise. For each question, ask a different group to provide their answer first. Ask all groups for any additional or differing interpretations and ideas. Encourage the students to discuss any disagreements. Return to the data if necessary.

4. Session conclusion and commitment to change (10 minutes): learners should be asked how they might make use of the data in their own practices. Ask them to commit to making just one change over this next year in relation to use of data in their evidence-based practice.

Resources

Agency for Health Care Quality and Research: http://www.ahrq.gov/qual/measurix.htm. On this website, you will find two reports: 1) the annual National Healthcare Disparities Reports (NHDR) examining the distribution of improvement in healthcare quality; and 2) the National Healthcare Quality Report (NHQR), addressing the current state of healthcare quality.

California Center for Health Statistics: http://www.dhs.ca.gov/hisp/chs/OHIR/reports/. This site provides a wide variety of data reports related to the health status of Californians. Of particular interest are the annual County Health Status Profiles that provide comparative data for all California counties in relation to each other and to the *Healthy People 2010* goals. Other data include deaths by zip code, and statistics for many disease states and causes of death.

Centers for Disease Control Office of Minority Health: http://www.cdc.gov/omh/AboutUs/disparities.htm. Obtain data on health disparities at the Center for Disease Control.

DHHS Office of Minority Health Resource Center: http://www.omhrc.gov/. This site has information in three categories: staying healthy, health disparities and communities in action.

Healthy People 2010: http://www.healthypeople.gov/Document/tableofcontents.htm. *Healthy People 2010* provides a large set of health objectives for the nation to achieve by the year 2010. The *Healthy People Midcourse Review* reports progress toward meeting the *Healthy People 2010* goals http://www.healthypeople.gov/data/midcourse/default.htm#pubs

Kaiser Family Foundation – State Health Facts: http://www.statehealthfacts.org/cgi-bin/healthfacts.cgi This site provides free, up-to-date, and easy-to-use health data on over 500 health topics for all 50 states.

National Center for Health Statistics: www.cdc.gov/nchs/data/hus/hus06.pdf. Health, United States 2006, with Chartbook on Trends in the Health of Americans provides data for the United States on a wide variety of health topics and provides comparisons including those by race, ethnicity, gender, and age. Downloads as a PDF document.

SESSIONS 8, 18 AND 28 Focused Review of Local, State, and National Health Data

Selecting Topics for Data Review

Potential Topics

1. Leading causes of death (http://www.cdc.gov/nchs/fastats/deaths.htm)
   Number of deaths for leading causes of death in the United States in 2005:
   Heart disease: 652,091
   Cancer: 559,312
   Stroke (cerebrovascular diseases): 143,579
   Chronic lower respiratory diseases: 130,933
   Accidents (unintentional injuries): 117,809
   Diabetes: 75,119
   Alzheimer's disease: 71,599
   Influenza/pneumonia: 63,001
   Nephritis, nephrotic syndrome, and nephrosis: 43,901
   Septicemia: 34,136
2. Topics within *Healthy People 2010*: Access and Medical Topics: http://www.healthypeople.gov/Document/tableofcontents.htm
3. Leading Health Indicators – *Healthy People 2010* tracks a group of leading health indicators that include: physical activity, overweight and obesity, tobacco use, substance abuse, responsible sexual behavior, mental health, injury and violence, environmental quality, and immunization. The Leading Health Indicators were selected on the basis of their 'ability to motivate action, the availability of data to measure progress, and their importance as public health issues.' http://www.healthypeople.gov/LHI/lhiwhat.htm
4. Access to Health Care Areas reported in state level reports. In the annual California County Health Status Profiles, mortality statistics are provided in the following areas: all causes of death, motor vehicle crashes, unintentional injuries, firearm injuries, homicide, suicide, all cancer deaths, lung cancer, female breast cancer, coronary heart disease, cerebrovascular disease (stroke), drug-induced deaths, and diabetes. http://www.dhs.ca.gov/hisp/chs/OHIR/reports/healthstatusprofiles/default.htm
5. The three areas we are suggesting are: 1. injuries and violence (a leading health indicator), 2. infant mortality and early pregnancy care, 3. diseases from among those where both state and national data are available (could have one for each small group among those most prevalent in your community).

Focused Review of Local, State, and National Health Data (Accidents, Homicide, and Suicide)

Sample Small Group Assignment with Data Sources

Directions: emergency rooms in Los Angeles County have been closing over the past 10 years. In 2007 there were only four level 3 and seven level 2 trauma centers listed for Los Angeles County. Is the need less now then it was in the year 2000? Look at the data in the areas of accidents and violence, and answer the following questions.

1. According the 2006 County Health Status Profiles for the state of California, how well is Los Angeles county doing in relation to other counties in the areas of:
   Motor vehicle crashes (pages 5–6)
   Unintentional injuries (pages 7–8)
   Firearm injuries (pages 9–10)
   Homicides (pages 11–12)
   Suicides (pages 13–14)?

2. Examine the statistics from the year 2000 (*2000 County Health Status Profile*) for the same topics (same page numbers as 2006). Which areas, if any, show improvement? How did you determine that?

3. Look further in the National Center for Health Statistics, *Health, United States 2006 with Chartbook on Trends in the Health of Americans* for the areas of homicides (Table 45, pages 227–9) and suicides (Table 46, pages 230–2). What are the differences, if any, by ethnicity/race among the groups nationally? In California? In the hospital/clinic (if data available)? Objectives 15–32 and 18–21 at: http://www.dhs.ca.gov/chs/OHIR/hp2010/hc2010progress.htm

4. Returning to our original issue of emergency facilities – think about how the absence of these facilities in certain areas could add to health care disparities through unequal access. Is this happening? How can you find out? List the additional data that would be required for you to understand the problem of equitable access to Emergency Care (or even more specifically, Trauma Care) in Los Angeles County.

SESSION 9 Annual Second Year Resident Patient Case Presentations: Cultural Issues in Negotiated Care

Session Description

This annual session (sessions 9, 19, and 29) is an application and integration exercise for second year residents to use the materials learned in the cultural competence curriculum up to this point. (With other learners this activity would be non-repeating and occur at the end of Unit V). The 'expanded case' format is used, with relevant cultural issues discussed. Each presenter will have prepared a brief description of a patient case where the patient's health beliefs were an issue in negotiating a care plan. The learner should demonstrate knowledge of the patient, and of any relevant historical model of health beliefs. Learners should be encouraged to include cases where alternative or ethno-medical healers were incorporated. Approximately five to seven learners can share within a one-hour session. Small groups with faculty group leaders can be used to allow more learners to present within a single session.

New in this session: this session introduces the teaching technique of 'expanded cases'. If it is unfamiliar to you, you may wish to review the relevant entry in Section 4.

Session Objectives

After participation in the session, learners should be better able to:
1. describe historical models of common health beliefs (for example, illness in the context of 'hot and cold'), and identify questions about health practices and beliefs that might be important in a specific local community (Objective 7 – knowledge)
2. identify healing traditions and beliefs of patients and their families, including ethno-medical beliefs, and describe (Objective 8 – skill)
3. describe models of effective cross-cultural communication, assessment, and physician–patient negotiation and identify common challenges in cross-cultural communication (for example, trust, style) (Objective 22 – knowledge)
4. assess and enhance patient adherence based on the patient's explanatory model. Describe ways to enhance patient adherence by collaborating with traditional and other community healers (Objective 25 – knowledge, skill).

Instructional Materials

Presentation assignment and guidelines, distributed some weeks prior to the presentation date to learners who will be presenting cases; materials requested by residents/students to facilitate case presentations; session objectives; commitment to change forms.

Time Schedule

00:00 – 00:03   Session introduction
00:03 – 00:45   Case presentations (maximum of seven six-minute case presentations)
00:45 – 00:55   Group discussion of common themes and session conclusion
00:55 – 01:00   Commitment to change

Process

Distribute presentation assignment and guidelines (attached) some weeks prior to the presentation date to learners who have been assigned to present cases. Instructors may want to review proposed cases with learners prior to the presentation date for appropriateness and relevance.
1. Introduction (3 minutes): this session requires only a brief introduction to present the session objectives to the learners, and explain how this session is part of the larger culturally responsive care curriculum.
2. Case presentations (42 minutes): each learner presents a case example of their work with a patient that illustrates culturally responsive care in terms of negotiating a culturally responsive treatment plan, incorporation of patient's health beliefs in treatment plan, as well as collaboration with alternative or ethno-medical healers. Relevant health outcomes should be mentioned.

3. Group discussion of common themes and session conclusion (10 minutes): use facilitation to engage all learners in discussion. Invite learners to identify any commonalities they observed in the case presentations in terms of clinical challenges and positive interventions.
4. Commitment to change (5 minutes): learners have the opportunity to write about their new learning based on the case presentations (both from preparing their own as well as listening to others). Encourage learners to commit to take one lesson directly back into their work.

Cautionary Note

Once learners begin this project, they will be challenged to keep their presentation brief and focused on the cultural aspects of the case. They may require guidance in pulling together relevant data instead of potentially presenting typical history and physical exam data, which may not be relevant to the task at hand.

Instructor Note

This exercise could easily be expanded into 30 minutes per learner, if time permits in your curriculum. Each learner presentation would be 20 minutes with 10 minutes for discussion. The presentation outline might be as follows: 1. case presentation; 2. formal discussion of the health belief system held by the patient; 3. a brief description of the cross-cultural communication model used by the resident; and 4. personal insights gained by the resident in the exploration of the case. Learners might use a PowerPoint presentation format to share their information with the group. Each presentation would be followed by discussion. The other learners should complete a formal evaluation of each of these presentations to assist the presenter in honing presentation skills.

Resources

Aberegg SK, Terry PB. Medical decision-making and healthcare disparities: the physician's role. *J Lab Clin Med*. 2004 Jul; **144**(1): 11–17.

Balsa AI, Seiler N, McGuire TG, *et al*. Clinical uncertainty and healthcare disparities. *Am J Law Med*. 2003; **29**(2–3): 203–19.

Lu FG, Lim R, Mezzich JE. Issues in the assessment and diagnosis of culturally diverse individuals. In: Oldham J and Riba M, editors. *Review of Psychiatry*, Vol. 14. Washington DC: American Psychiatric Press; 1995: 477–510.

Thiel de Bocanegra H, Gany F. Good provider, good patient: changing behaviors to eliminate disparities in healthcare. *Am J Manag Care*. 2004 Sep; **10** Spec No: SP20–8.

SESSION 9 – RESIDENT HANDOUT Cultural Medicine Case Presentation Preparation Guidelines

You are to prepare a six-minute presentation of a case that illustrates your culturally responsive work with a patient. The presentation will be on (insert date here), and you will be one of (insert number) presenters that day.

Objectives

The objectives of these presentations are to:

1. describe the patient's historical model of health belief (if applicable) and the questions about health practices and beliefs that were important to your understanding of that patient's model
2. identify healing traditions and beliefs of patients and their families, including ethno-medical beliefs and use of ethno-medical healers
3. describe any model of cross-cultural communication, assessment, and physician–patient negotiation that you used and identify any challenges you faced (for example, trust, style)
4. if appropriate, describe how you worked to enhance patient adherence by collaborating with traditional and other community healers.

Instructions

1. Select a case where a health belief of the patient was relevant to your care. You should be able to discuss the health belief in the context of any relevant historical model of health care belief. In selecting your case, pick one where negotiation of a care plan that incorporated the patient's health beliefs was important and/or where collaboration with alternative or ethno-medical healers took place.
2. You may discuss your case selection with the course instructor in terms of appropriateness and relevance of the case to the cultural medicine curriculum and session goals.
3. Given the brief time allotted for the presentation, be very judicious in selecting which aspects of the case to include. For example, share only case history data that directly apply to the health belief in question, use of alternative/complementary medicine, and any cultural negotiation of the treatment plan.
4. Be sure to share insights you have gained about the health belief in question from research you did on that belief.
5. Practice your presentation – six minutes is brief, so timing is important.

SESSION 10 Annual Review of Individual Cultural Competency Commitments

Session Description

The final session in each year of the three-year curriculum (sessions 10, 20 and 30) provides an opportunity for learners to use reflection and self-assessment to contemplate their set of commitments to change and their progress to date. Learners will be provided the opportunity to share with each other, if they so chose, some of their areas of positive growth, as well as remaining challenges. There will also be time for general discussion in relation to ways for reducing bias of the providers and for addressing disparities for patients within their practice environment. The group might select one thing to work on over the next academic year. In the second and third year, the group should spend some time in this session discussing progress over the past year on their target goal.

New in this session: this session introduces two teaching methods, 'reflection and self-assessment' and 'portfolio', described in Section 4.

Session Objectives

After participation in the session, learners should be better able to:
1. become aware of their own cultural heritage, gender, class, ethnic-racial identity, sexual orientation, disability, age and spirituality; reflect on it and describe it (Objective 2 – awareness, skill)
2. recognize their own potential for bias and stereotyping, identify their own stereotypes and biases and explore how their attitudes, biases and stereotypes affect clinical encounters, clinical decision-making and quality of care (Objective 12 – awareness, knowledge)
3. describe strategies for reducing physician's own biases, and those of others, and demonstrate strategies to assess, manage, and reduce bias and its effects in the clinical encounter and in clinical practice (Objective 15 – skill)
4. describe patterns of health care disparities that can result, at least in part, from physician bias, recognize disparities that are amenable to intervention, and value eliminating disparities. (Objective 20 – attitude, knowledge).

Instructional Materials

Flip chart and pens; the entire set of objectives for the Cultural Competence Curriculum for review; collected learner materials for each learner (presentations, quizzes, reflective writings, commitments to change, etc.), which should be distributed to each learner at the start of the session.

Time Schedule

00:00 – 00:05   Session introduction
00:05 – 00:20   Independent review of journal, reflections and commitments
00:20 – 00:40   Open discussion
00:40 – 00:55   Plan for change, think-pair-share
00:55 – 01:00   Session conclusion

Process

1. Introduction (5 minutes): this session requires only a brief introduction to the importance of this session as part of the larger culturally responsive care curriculum.
2. Independent review (15 minutes): learners are provided with their complete set of materials collected over the course of their participation in the cultural medicine curriculum (including orientation materials for first-year residents). Ask them to review the materials with an eye to their positive growth, areas for further and future growth, the degree to which they have been able to fulfill their commitments, and any barriers faced in fulfilling those commitments. Learners may wish to highlight outstanding learning experiences and/or clinical encounters over the past year.

3. Open discussion (20 minutes): here the group is invited to share their findings from the independent review (described above). Successes, frustrations, and barriers can be highlighted by the group facilitator on flip charts at the front of the room. A revisiting of the Cultural Curriculum objectives can be helpful and included as part of this discussion. The skills of facilitation will help ensure a student-centered discussion.
4. Plan for change/think-write-share (15 minutes): looking to the future, learners are asked to write their personal goals for professional growth toward culturally responsive care, including any personal areas of bias, stereotyping, and/or discomfort. Next, each learner shares these with a partner, and finally the group as a whole joins a larger discussion of future learning goals.
5. Session conclusion (5 minutes): this is an opportunity to thank the learners for their input today and over this segment of the curriculum (Sessions A, B, C and 1–10) and remind them that the curriculum uses a spiral model. In the next year, the learners will revisit each of the six units, and again in the third year of the curriculum.

Instructor Note

Learners often have a tendency to focus more on the negative than the positive in their own professional trajectory. It is important that the facilitator help learners share both frustrations and observed areas of growth and accomplishment in a balanced fashion.

Resources

Betancourt JR. Cultural competence and medical education: many names, many perspectives, one goal. *Acad Med.* 2006 Jun; **81**(6): 499–501.

Chambers N. Close encounters: the use of critical reflective analysis as an evaluation tool in teaching and learning. *J Adv Nurs.* 1999; **29**(4): 950–7.

Like RC. Culturally competent family medicine: transforming clinical practice and ourselves. *Am Fam Physician. 2005 Dec;* **72**(11): 2189.

Murray-Garcia JL, Harrell S, Garcia JA, *et al.* Self-reflection in multicultural training: be careful what you ask for. *Acad Med.* 2005 Jul; **80**(7): 694–701.

SESSION 11 Bias, Communication, and Quality

Session Description

This session introduces the second year of the curriculum and may be the first session beyond the orientation sessions for some learners. It serves to facilitate exploration of the clinician's personal experiences of being different from others. It also explores their reactions to patients and how these are potentially linked to the quality of care provided. The learners are encouraged to discover and articulate their own personal vulnerabilities to providing lesser care to some patients, which can contribute to health care disparities. The session concludes with commitment to change.

New in this session: this session introduces the exercise, 'drawing differences', described in Section 5. If it is unfamiliar to you, you may wish to review the relevant entry.

Session Objectives

After participation in the session, learners should be better able to:

1. define, in contemporary terms, race, ethnicity, and culture (Objective 1 – knowledge)
2. recognize their own potential for bias and stereotyping, be able to identify their own stereotypes and biases, and explore how their attitudes, biases and stereotypes affect clinical encounters, clinical decision-making and quality of care (Objective 12 – awareness, knowledge)
3. identify and appreciate how clinician bias and stereotyping can affect interactions with patients, families, communities, and other members of the health care team, and the link between effective communication and quality care (Objective 13 – attitude, knowledge)
4. describe systemic and medical-encounter issues related to health care disparities, including communication issues, clinical decision-making, and patient preferences (Objective 21 – knowledge).

Instructional Materials

Art supplies for the 'drawing differences' exercise including crayons and paper; flip chart and pens; instructions for small group exercise; materials for commitment to change.

Time Schedule

00:00 – 00:10   Session introduction and drawing differences exercise
00:10 – 00:25   Debriefing of exercise
00:25 – 00:40   Small group exercise
00:40 – 00:55   Large group discussion
00:55 – 01:00   Commitment to change

Process

1. Session introduction (10 minutes): the session opens with an exercise called drawing differences (*see* Section 5 for details). Each learner is provided with a piece of paper and a crayon or two. They are invited to close their eyes and the facilitator recites the following instructions:

   Think about a time in your life when you felt different in some way. It may be the first time that you felt different from others. As best you can, picture the situation including where you were, who you were with, and any feelings associated with the experience of difference.

   Learners are given a minute or two in silence to conjure the memory. Next they are instructed to capture that memory of difference in a crayon drawing. The drawing is done in silence and typically takes about five minutes.
   When the learners are done drawing, share the session objectives with them.
2. Debriefing (15 minutes): open the debriefing by asking each learner to share his/her drawing and the experience it portrays with a partner (5 minutes). Ask the pairs to share drawings

and stories of difference with the group (5 minutes). In large group sharing, the instructor records two columns of information in front of the group: 1. types of differences and 2. the feelings associated with the experience of those differences. When the group looks at the list of experiences, ask for any general conclusions in relation to feeling different – generally learners comment that most of the experiences were negative, and that many memories of 'first' experiences happened when young (5 minutes).

3. Small group exercise and sharing of results (15 minutes): place the learners in small groups. Provide the following instructions for an exercise on how patients and providers differ (handout attached):

   a) *Quickly list the ways that your patients may differ from you – don't judge each other's ideas, just record them.* (Instructor: these should be very long lists – e.g. gender, age, ethnicity, religion, emotional and intellectual capability, educational level, musical or artistic talent, background, disability, sexual orientation, life experiences [abuse, neglect, loss, violence, prison, homelessness, etc.], personality, interaction style, spiritual beliefs, physical appearance, state of health, marital status, parental status, hygiene, mental status.)

   b) *Pick two items from the list that at least one person in the group finds challenging for him/her in providing excellent care (e.g., hygiene, emotionality). Provide your ideas about why each difference provides a challenge and how it might affect care.* (Instructor: it does not matter what they selected – the focus is on thoughtful reflection as to impacts on the provider/patient relationship.)

   The first challenge should take about two minutes, leaving eight minutes for the second. Monitor the small groups to ensure that they are on task. The final five minutes should be reserved for sharing results. Spend this entire time on having each group share one answer to the second challenge.

4. Discussion (15 minutes): post the definitions of stereotype, prejudice and discrimination (one set of these can be found at www.tolerance.org in the Primer on Hidden Bias). Think together about how discrimination can contribute to health care disparities and what we can do to monitor ourselves to avoid it.

5. Commitment to change (5 minutes): forms or cards are filled out, including an identification of at least two biases/challenging patient characteristics the learner hopes to grow more adept at navigating.

Cautionary Notes

1. This is a very important session in terms of helping learners face the often unexpressed experience of personal discomfort with patients, types of patients, certain health conditions and, perhaps ethnic, gender, sexual orientation aspects of certain groups of patients.

2. For students/residents that have not yet visited key self-reflection websites, you can recommend the PBS Race website, the IAT website, and the Primer on Hidden Bias at www.tolerance.org.

Resources

Implicit Association Test (IAT): https://implicit.harvard.edu/implicit/demo/

Johnson RL, Saha S, Arbelaez JJ, *et al.* Racial and ethnic differences in patient perceptions of bias and cultural competence in health care. *J Gen Intern Med.* 2004 Feb; **19**(2): 101–10.

National Healthcare Disparity Reports produced each year by AHRQ. Available from: http://www.ahrq.gov/qual/measurix.htm

Race – The Power of an Illusion. PBS Race Website: http://www.pbs.org/race

Schulman KA, Berlin JA, Harless W, *et al.* The effect of race and sex on physicians' recommendations for cardiac catheterization. *N Eng J Med.* 1999 Feb 25; **340**(8): 618–26.

Smedley BD, Stith AY, Nelson AR, editors. *Unequal Treatment: Confronting Racial and Ethnic Disparities in Health Care.* Board on Health Sciences Policy. Washington, DC: National Academies Press; 2002. Available from: http://www.iom.edu/CMS/3740/4475.aspx

Tolerance.org (Southern Poverty Law Center): http://www.tolerance.org/index.jsp

SESSION 11 Bias, Communication and Quality

Small Group Exercise

The ability to distinguish friend from foe helped early humans survive, and the ability to quickly and automatically categorize people is a fundamental quality of the human mind. Categories give order to life, and every day, we group other people into categories based on social and other characteristics. This is the foundation of stereotypes, prejudice and, ultimately, discrimination.

Tolerance.org, Hidden Bias: A Primer.

Directions: Select a recorder. Use the flip chart (or giant Post-a-Note pad) to record your responses.
1. Quickly list the ways that your patients may differ from you – don't judge each other's ideas, just record them.
2. Select two of the above differences that at least one person in the group finds challenging for him/her in providing excellent care. Provide your ideas about why each difference provides a challenge and how it might affect care.

Difference 1
What makes this difference challenging in the clinical encounter?
List ways this could affect the care provided.

Difference 2
What makes this difference challenging in the clinical encounter?
List ways this could affect the care provided.

SESSION 12 Culturally Responsive Interview: Health Beliefs

Session Description

This session opens with the viewing of a cross-cultural video (*Worlds Apart* video, Justine Chitsena's story, *see* Video Resources in Section 7). The video clip displays a case of a multi-generational immigrant family where traditional beliefs and modern medicine clash. The discussion will provide the learners with several new tools that can be used to aid their inter-action with patients. The patient-oriented case portion of a tool called the 'SOAP Grid' will be reinforced in this session, while the interviewing mnemonic Q2 will be introduced. Q2 is two simple questions that can be asked of any patient in any visit to very briefly explore health beliefs. Role play will be used so that learners can practice using the tools. In this session the learners will also be provided with a handout that provides information about health beliefs that are common to various immigrant populations so that they are alert to beliefs that patients from these groups (or their family members) may hold. A learner journal of reflections and commitments to change will be begun in this session and continue to be used throughout the year.

New in this session: in this session we recommend introduction of learner journals as a technique to be used throughout this year. You may wish to review the relevant entry in Section 4.

Session Objectives

After participation in the session, learners should be better able to:
1. identify healing traditions and beliefs of patients and their families, including ethno-medical beliefs. Ask questions in a non-judgmental manner to elicit patient preferences, listen and respond appropriately to patient feedback about key cross-cultural issues. Elicit additional information about ethno-medical conditions and ethno-medical healers (Objective 8 – attitudes, knowledge, skill)
2. exhibit comfort when conversing with patients/colleagues about cultural issues (Objective 9 – attitudes)
3. conduct and document a culturally responsive history and physical examination within the context of family-centered care. Elicit a cultural, social, and medical history, including a patient's health beliefs/model of their illness (Objective 23 – skill).

Instructional Materials

Worlds Apart video clip, Justine Chitsena's story (first seven minutes only); VCR and projector; two role playing scenarios; a journal for each learner.

Time Schedule

00:00 – 00:05 Session introduction
00:05 – 00:13 Introduction of Q2 and review of Patient-Centered Care section of SOAP Grid
00:13 – 00:20 *Worlds Apart* Justine Chitsena video clip (first seven minutes only)
00:20 – 00:35 Review of the case discussing all relevant SOAP Grid questions
00:35 – 00:50 Role play using Q2
00:50 – 01:00 Conclusion: introduction to the use of a journal with commitment to change

Process

1. Introduction (5 minutes): as this session focuses on health beliefs, you might use a relevant opener to grab the learners' attention – a picture, a poem, a brief anecdote from practice should help set the tone.
2. Didactic presentation (8 minutes): this brief didactic presentation focuses on the importance of understanding a patient's world view when assessing a problem and in formulating a treatment plan. The Q2 mnemonic is based on the work of Arthur Kleinman. It is introduced here and consists of two simple questions: 'what do you think made you sick?' and 'what do you think could help you get better?'

3. Presentation of video clip (7 minutes): show the first seven minutes of the *Worlds Apart* video of the Justine Chitsena case, which highlights the impact of multi-generational family health beliefs on care planning. Instruct the learners to be thinking about the SOAP Grid questions as they view the video.

4. Discussion of Justine Chitsena as an expanded case (15 minutes): ask learners the questions in the Subjective box of the Patient-Centered section of the SOAP Grid (handout attached) and facilitate a discussion. The questions that have been indicated in bold typeface are thought to be the most appropriate in promoting a discussion about incorporating health beliefs in negotiated and patient-centered care. At the conclusion of the discussion, it is helpful to emphasize that mnemonics like Q2 (and HEADDSS, BATHE, ETHNIC) serve as a roadmap for navigating the patient encounter. It is incumbent on each learner to experiment with these strategies in the development of their own roadmap toward effective doctor–patient communication.

5. Role play process (15 minutes): have the Q2 mnemonic written in large letters at the front of the meeting room. Divide learners into pairs, one who will take the role of patient, the other of doctor. Have them move their chairs so that they face each other, but that the learner in the doctor role faces the mnemonic posted at the front.

   a) Ask the learner playing the patient to think of a real patient they have worked with, and to be that patient for the exercise (or provide your own case). Review the following process with the learners. The entire interchange should take approximately 5 minutes:

   Doctor: begins by welcoming the patient and inquiring as to what brings him/her in.
   Patient: briefly (one or two sentences) describes a problem.
   Doctor: inquires more about the problem via the Q2 mnemonic.

   b) Reverse roles using the second case.
   c) Debrief: first ask learners about the role of the doctor and to comment on what went well in the exercise, and/or what new learning they acquired. Next, ask them to comment on difficulties or challenges. This is followed by feedback from the 'patient' point of view about positive (first) and then any problematic perceptions of the encounter. Learners can be challenged to begin to consider how they might negotiate a treatment plan incorporating both patient health beliefs and the medical perspective (knowledge, experience, evidence).

6. Journal and commitment to change (10 minutes): introduce the concept of the journal as a convenient way to keep track of their commitments over this next year. Distribute a journal to each learner and have learners complete the first entry – a commitment to change related to this session expressing at least one thing they will do differently in their care of patients based on what they learned in this session.

Resource

Kleinman A. *The Illness Narratives: Suffering, healing, and the human condition*. New York: Basic Books; 1988.
Levin SJ, Like RC, Gottlieb JC. Useful clinical interviewing mnemonics. *Patient Care*. 2000; **34**: 189–90.

SESSION 12 Cultural Competence SOAP Grid

Patient-Centered Care Portion Adapted for Justine Chitsena case

The CC SOAP Grid was designed to offer a number of 'onramps' to discussion of cultural issues in a typical patient case. The body of the grid is comprised of specific questions for the resident/student regarding the subjective, objective, assessment, and plan components of a case. There is also an additional row entitled post-hoc reflection that provides a number of 'big picture' follow-up questions about culture and patient care.

Here the patient-centered care portion of the grid has been modified for use in reviewing the care provided by another clinician. The entire grid with directions can be found in Section 6.

Subjective	**Did the physician ask about the patient's health beliefs (Q2)?**
	What parts of the patient's story require follow up in the next visit?
Objective	Did you feel uncomfortable at any time while conducting physical exam? How did it impact the exam? What should you do to grow from this experience?
	Did the patient appear uncomfortable during your exam? If so, how did you address the patient's feelings?
Assessment	Did the assessment/problem list address the patient's reasons for coming to the clinic?
	Did the patient/parent understand and agree with the assessment and how do you know?
	Are there any discrepancies between the assessment and the patient's health belief system? Please describe.
Plan	**Are there any concerns about the patient's/parent's ability or willingness to adhere to the treatment plan, and how could you negotiate issues with the patient?**
	How could you address the grandmother's culturally based concerns regarding the treatment plan?
	Assuming the assessment is correct, how would you proceed in order to negotiate a culturally acceptable and medically sound plan?
Post-Hoc Reflection	What is your plan to become more knowledgeable and skillful in regard to this patient's special population?
	What went well and what did not work in your negotiation with this patient?
	How can models with acronyms like Q2, ETHNIC, and LEARN assist you in your care of patients?

SESSION 13 Cultural Knowledge: Discussion of a Selected Cultural Group

Session Description

Three sessions (sessions 3, 13, and 23) are designated as annual cultural knowledge sessions. Session 13 is designed to include multiple brief student/resident presentations. Health professions students and residents do an excellent job in developing these types of presentation. The intent is for the local program to select one or more areas of interest, preferably cultural groups that, while present in the greater community, are not part of the clinical practice of the learners. Quickfact sheets can be obtained for any state or county and many major cities. In addition to groups selected by country or ethnicity, religious groups could also be the focus for a session, again selected to enlarge the knowledge base of the learners.

Session Objectives

After participation in the session, learners should be better able to:
1. value the importance of diversity in health care and address the challenges and opportunities it poses (Objective 3 – attitude)
2. describe historical models of common health beliefs (for example, illness in the context of 'hot and cold') and identify questions about health practices and beliefs that might be important in a specific local community (Objective 7 – knowledge)
3. discuss race, ethnicity, and culture in the context of the medical interview and health care. Exhibit comfort when conversing with patients/colleagues about cultural issues (Objective 9 – attitude, skill)
4. describe methods to identify key community leaders. Describe strategies for partnering with community activists to eliminate racism and other bias from health care. Collaborate to address community needs (Objective 28 – knowledge, skill).

Instructional Materials

Presentation outline, distributed some weeks prior to the presentation date if learners will be presenting cases, or used to guide the faculty's development of the session; materials requested by learners to facilitate presentations (a list of potential resources is provided); session objectives; small group activity; journal.

Time Schedule

00:00 – 00:15   Introductory activity (interview with community member or leader, video clip, panel, quiz/trivia contest, case presentation, etc. – *see* openers in Section 4)

00:15 – 00:45   Formal presentation of information from individual learners or pairs (5–8 minutes each)

00:45 – 00:55   Group discussion in relation to a) implications for care of patients; b) community resources; and c) how learners might collaborate with community leaders to address needs of groups discussed

00:55 – 01:00   Session summary and journal

Process

Distribute presentation assignment and guidelines (*see* attached) some weeks prior to the presentation date if learners will be assigned to prepare for this session. Instructors will want to work with any group of learners in preparing their presentation, particularly if this is their first experience.

1. Introductory activity (15 minutes): the initial stimulus material or introductory activity (opener) should engage the audience and introduce the topic and may last from 5 to 15 minutes. Potential methods include: interview with community member or leader, video clip/debriefing, panel, quiz/trivia contest (using teams, audience response system, or paper and pencil), case presentation, etc. In the Video Resources section (Section 7) there are several sources that provide relevant clips including brief segments from the *Worlds Apart*

tapes (Laotian child, African-American man, Mexican-American woman, and Muslim man). Caution: if a video is used it should focus the audience on the objectives for this session.

2. Formal learner presentations of information (30 minutes): the formal presentation of information can be done using PowerPoint or can be provided in a handout. PowerPoint allows insertion of a short video clip, photograph, quiz, etc., for the audience. *See* the attached outline for an overview of the materials to cover if the focus is a cultural group (e.g. African-Americans, Hispanics), people from a specific country (e.g. Mexico, China); or a specific religious heritage (e.g. Muslim, Buddhist). Each learner or pair of learners would get 5–8 minutes to share some of the health beliefs of a specific group.

4. Small group discussion (10 minutes): select one of the following topics for a focused discussion with the learners: a) implications of the culturally based health beliefs for care of patients; b) community resources for cultural groups presented; and c) how learners might collaborate with community leaders to address needs for an identified group.

5. Conclusion and journal (5 minutes): the instructor should thank the learners that presented and request that each learner (presenters and audience) write an entry into his/her journal that reflects a commitment to take new learning directly back into their clinical work or into their participation in the health center or community.

Cautionary Note

It is important to emphasize that knowledge learning about other groups helps health care providers develop hypotheses about the cultural background of patients. In the end, providers must strive to hold stereotyping 'at bay' and draw conclusions based on information provided by the patient himself/herself.

SESSION 13 HANDOUT: Cultural Knowledge Presentation Preparation Guidelines

Directions: This session focuses on cultural knowledge. You can select a cultural group, a specific country or a religious group for your brief presentation. For the group selected conduct research. A list of resources is attached. Plan and rehearse a formal presentation (5–8 minutes). You may want to provide a handout or to prepare a brief PowerPoint presentation. If using PowerPoint try to include visual images to enhance the presentation. Use no more than 5–8 slides. The presentation should focus on the things most relevant to health beliefs or on health and health care disparities. The talk might be divided into two parts with more time spent on the last sections.

Overview (1–3 minutes)
1. *Country* – language, including number of dialects; any important interpersonal relationships (e.g., naming, status, roles, greetings, displays of respect, general etiquette); unique information about marriage, family kinship (marriage, gender roles, extended families); religious beliefs and practices.
2. *Ethnic Group* – same information as for 'country' with addition of countries of origin.
3. *Religious Group* – basic tenants in relevant areas of daily living.

Health beliefs and practices (4–5 minutes)
Described in general or in relation to relevant topics like: a) reproduction (pregnancy, child birth, post partum practices); b) nutrition and food; c) alcohol, drugs, tobacco; d) attitudes toward death and suffering; e) complementary therapies.

Or

Disparities and community resources (4–5 minutes)
Discuss any data on health disparities in your community, state, or in the nation and provide information about local community leader(s) and community groups/resources serving this community.

SESSION 13 Cultural Knowledge

Web-Based Resources

A wide variety of health care and educational institutions have websites that provide information about various cultures, religions and other minority groups. The following websites can be used both for this presentation as well as for enhancing medical care to unfamiliar groups.

http://bearspace.baylor.edu/Charles_Kemp/www/refugees.htm
This site provides resources for cross-cultural care and prevention in relation to a variety of Asian cultures including Burmese, Cambodian/Khmer, Laotian/Lao, Vietnamese, Indian (Asian), as well as information on refugee and immigrant health.

http://www.beliefnet.com/
This site provides useful neutrally written descriptions of 28 different faiths and their belief structures, including Buddhism, Hinduism, Christianity (many variants), Islam, Judaism, Pagan and earth-based Taoism, and Sikhism.

http://www.ethnomed.org/
This site contains culture specific pages as well as pages on cross cultural health topics. The University of Washington maintains the site. The site evolves but cultural profiles for the following cultural groups: Cambodian, Chinese, Eritrean, Ethiopian (also Oromo and Tigrean people), Hmong, Mexican, Somali, and Vietnamese.

http://www.health.qld.gov.au/multicultural/health_workers/cultdiver_guide.asp
This site provides information about the following cultural groups from the perspective of the health care system in Queensland, Australia: Bosnian Muslims, Cambodians, Chinese, Croatians, Greeks, Hmong, Italians, Muslims from West Asia, Philippines, Samoans, Tongans, Serbians, and Vietnamese.

http://www.healthsystem.virginia.edu/internet/chaplaincy/
This site provides brief helpful descriptions of Buddhism, Hinduism, Islam, Christianity (Protestant, Catholic) and Judaism. It provides a booklet *Religious Beliefs and Practices Affecting Health Care* developed for use by UVA Health System staff. Hard copies of the booklet are also available for $3/copy or $30/dozen. The PDF file is also available for $25 and allows the purchaser to make and distribute copies at their own institution.

http://www.hispanichealth.org/
This site has resources for purchase including: *Delivering Health Care to Hispanics: A manual for providers.* 3rd ed. (2004) and the Companion Workbook; and *A Primer for Cultural Proficiency: Towards quality health services for Hispanics* (2001).

http://www.metrokc.gov/health/glbt/
These web pages address the health concerns of gay, lesbian, bisexual, and transgender people, also known as 'GLBT' people and 'sexual minorities'.

SESSION 14 Institutional Self-Reflection on Cultural Competence and CLAS (Culturally and Linguistically Appropriate Services) Standards

Session Description

Standard 9 of the CLAS Standards states 'Health care organizations should conduct initial and ongoing organizational self-assessments of CLAS-related activities and are encouraged to integrate cultural and linguistic competence-related measures into their internal audits, performance improvement programs, patient satisfaction assessments, and outcomes-based evaluations.' This session provides an opportunity for just this type of self-reflection on the medical institution where the learners do their work and/or study.

Session Objectives

After participation in this session, learners should be better able to:
1. value the importance of diversity in health care and address the challenges and opportunities it poses (Objective 3 – attitude)
2. recognize and describe institutional cultural issues for own institution and discuss the CLAS Standards (Objective 10 – knowledge)
3. review and discuss the CLAS Standards, institutional challenges related to health care disparities, and strategies for using the CLAS standards as a tool to address disparities (Objective 21 – knowledge).

Instructional Materials

CLAS Standards handout (attached); small group assignment handouts; flip charts and markers for small group presentations; DVD or online connection/projection for A Physician's Practical Guide to Culturally Competent Care at www.thinkculturalhealth.org (optional); post-test on the CLAS Standards (optional).

Time Schedule

00:00 – 00:05   Session introduction
00:05 – 00:10   Provide an overview of the CLAS Standards
00:10 – 00:25   Small group activity – assessing our organization in relation to CLAS
00:25 – 00:40   Small group presentations to the larger group
00:40 – 00:55   Facilitation of general discussion of the organization's culture and how to enhance cultural competence and quality
00:55 – 01:00   Session conclusion and journal

Process

1. Session introduction (5 minutes): this session might begin with a poll of learners as an opener: 'how many of you have provided care for a patient whose native language was different from yours?' Note the number or percent of the group. Then using the flip chart list language challenges than can be faced when providing care.
2. Overview of CLAS Standards (5 minutes): distribute the CLAS Standards and provide a brief presentation of the history of the development of the CLAS Standards, how they are organized into themes and a brief discussion of mandates versus guidelines versus recommendations.
3. Small group activity (15 minutes): divide participants into three groups (more if group is larger than 24) and assign one of the themes within the CLAS Standards to each group. Instruct learners to assess how well your organization (clinic, hospital) is doing in relation to the assigned theme, including strengths and weaknesses. They should be prepared to share their assessment along with their ideas for how the institution could improve in relation to their theme. Each group should be provided with a flip chart and markers to facilitate their thinking, organization, and ultimate presentation, and will need to select a spokesperson for the presentation. Group sizes can range from three to eight participants. Each group

should be provided with a handout (attached) listing their assigned CLAS Standards and a guide for their discussion and presentation.

4. Small group presentations (15 minutes): each group will briefly a) describe the theme they were assigned; b) discuss the institution's strengths and weaknesses in relation to the theme; and c) present strategies that could be used to move toward successful implementation of the set of Standards.

5. Group discussion – beyond the standards (15 minutes): facilitate a discussion with the group about the culture of the institution. What are its primary characteristics? In its daily functioning, what things encourage and what things discourage physicians, other health care professionals and the staff from acting in a culturally competent manner? Finally, list ideas for how each current or future provider can act to move the medical institutional culture forward toward excellence in this area.

6. Journal and session conclusion (5 minutes): conclude with each learner writing one important take-home message into his/her journal. Alternatively, a brief post-test on general knowledge of the CLAS Standards might be developed and administered.

Instructor Note

If the group is very large, the instructor may wish to simply divide the group in thirds and have them work in pairs (think-pair-share) on their assigned theme. *See* attached assignment. Also, you may want to have several hospital resource people at the session to answer learner questions in relation to each 'theme' as they conduct their assessments. Be sure to advise representatives that their role is merely to provide data, not to defend the institution.

Resources

Anderson LM, Scrimshaw SC, Fullilove MT, *et al.* Task Force on Community Preventive Services. Culturally competent healthcare systems: a systematic review. *Am J Prev Med.* 2003; **24**(3 Suppl): 68–79.

Bender DE, Clawson M, Harlan C, *et al.* Improving access for Latino immigrants: evaluation of language training adapted to the needs of health professionals. *J Immigrant Health.* 2004; **6**(4): 197–209.

The CLAS Standards. Available from: www.omhrc.gov

Kairys JA, Like RC. Caring for diverse populations: do academic family medicine practices have CLAS? *Fam Med.* 2006 Mar; **38**(3): 196–205.

Larson L. Is your hospital culturally competent? (And what does that mean exactly?). *Trustee.* 2005 Feb; **58**(2): 20–3, 3.

Minkler M, ed. *Community Organizing and Community Building for Health.* New Jersey: The Rutgers State University; 1999.

Narayan MC. The national standards for culturally and linguistically appropriate services in health care. *Care Manag J.* 2001–2002 Winter; **3**(2): 77–83.

A Physician's Practical Guide to Culturally Competent Care. Available from: www.thinkculturalhealth.org

Rhyne R, Bogue R, Kukulka G, *et al.*, editors. *Community-Oriented Primary Care: Health care for the 21st century.* Washington DC: American Public Health Association; 1998.

Salimbene S. *CLAS A–Z: A Practical Guide for Implementing the National Standards for Culturally and Linguistically Appropriate Services (CLAS) in Health Care.* Rockford, IL: Inter-Face International; 2002. Available from: http://www.omhrc.gov/templates/browse.aspx?lvl=1&lvlID=13

SESSION 14 National Standards for Culturally and Linguistically Appropriate Services (CLAS)

The CLAS Standards are primarily directed at health care organizations; however, individual providers are also encouraged to use the standards to make their practices more culturally and linguistically accessible. The principles and activities of culturally and linguistically appropriate services should be integrated throughout an organization and undertaken in partnership with the communities being served. The 14 standards are organized by themes: Culturally Competent Care (Standards 1–3), Language Access Services (Standards 4–7), and Organizational Supports for Cultural Competence (Standards 8–14). Within this framework, there are three types of standards of varying stringency: mandates, guidelines, and recommendations as follows:

CLAS **mandates** are current Federal requirements for all recipients of Federal funds (Standards 4, 5, 6, and 7). CLAS **guidelines** are activities recommended by the Office of Minority Health (OMH) for adoption as mandates by Federal, State, and National accrediting agencies (Standards 1, 2, 3, 8, 9, 10, 11, 12, and 13). CLAS **recommendations** are suggested by OMH for voluntary adoption by health care organizations (Standard 14).

Standard 1
Health care organizations should ensure that patients/consumers receive from all staff members effective, understandable, and respectful care that is provided in a manner compatible with their cultural health beliefs and practices and preferred language.

Standard 2
Health care organizations should implement strategies to recruit, retain, and promote at all levels of the organization a diverse staff and leadership that are representative of the demographic characteristics of the service area.

Standard 3
Health care organizations should ensure that staff at all levels and across all disciplines receive ongoing education and training in culturally and linguistically appropriate service delivery.

Standard 4
Health care organizations must offer and provide language assistance services, including bilingual staff and interpreter services, at no cost to each patient/consumer with limited English proficiency at all points of contact, in a timely manner, during all hours of operation.

Standard 5
Health care organizations must provide to patients/consumers in their preferred language both verbal offers and written notices informing them of their right to receive language assistance services.

Standard 6
Health care organizations must assure the competence of language assistance provided to patients/consumers with limited English proficiency by interpreters and bilingual staff. Family and friends should not be used to provide interpretation services (except on request by the patient/consumer).

Standard 7
Health care organizations must make available easily understood patient-related materials and post signage in the languages of the commonly encountered groups represented in the service area.

Standard 8
Health care organizations should develop, implement, and promote a written strategic plan that outlines clear goals, policies, operational plans, and management accountability/oversight mechanisms to provide culturally and linguistically appropriate services.

Standard 9

Health care organizations should conduct initial and ongoing organizational self-assessments of CLAS-related activities and are encouraged to integrate cultural and linguistic competence-related measures into their internal audits, performance improvement programs, patient satisfaction assessments, and outcomes-based evaluations.

Standard 10

Health care organizations should ensure that data on the individual patient's/consumer's race, ethnicity, and spoken and written language are collected in health records, integrated into the organization's management information systems, and periodically updated.

Standard 11

Health care organizations should maintain a current demographic, cultural, and epidemiological profile of the community as well as a needs assessment to accurately plan for and implement services that respond to the cultural and linguistic characteristics of the service area.

Standard 12

Health care organizations should develop participatory, collaborative partnerships with communities and utilize a variety of formal and informal mechanisms to facilitate community and patient/consumer involvement in designing and implementing CLAS-related activities.

Standard 13

Health care organizations should ensure that conflict and grievance resolution processes are culturally and linguistically sensitive and capable of identifying, preventing, and resolving cross-cultural conflicts or complaints by patients/consumers.

Standard 14

Health care organizations are encouraged to regularly make available to the public information about their progress and successful innovations in implementing the CLAS standards and to provide public notice in their communities about the availability of this information.

Content last modified: 10/17/2005, 6:30:00 PM
http://www.omhrc.gov/templates/browse.aspx?lvl=2@lvlID=15
Office of Minority Health, Department of Health and Human Services
Downloaded, 2008 July 4.

SESSION 14 Institutional Self-Reflection on Cultural Competence and CLAS Standards

Small Group Activity

Directions: review the set of standards for your group's assigned theme. Think about your clinic and hospital setting. List the strengths and weaknesses of it in relation to the theme. Brainstorm and record all of your ideas for institutional improvement in relation to your assigned theme. Pick several that you all agree upon. Be prepared to share your ideas with the other groups.

Theme 1 – Culturally Competent Care (Standards 1–3)
Theme 2 – Language Access Services (Standards 4–7)
Theme 3 – Organizational Supports for Cultural Competence (Standards 8–14)

Your Theme Number _____

Strengths	Weaknesses/Challenges	Ideas for Improvement

SESSION 14 Institutional Self-Reflection on Cultural Competence and CLAS Standards

Think-Pair-Share Activity for Groups Larger than 50

Directions: review the set of standards for your assigned theme. Think about your clinic and hospital setting. List the strengths and weaknesses in relation to the theme. Brainstorm and record all of your joint ideas for institutional improvement in relation to your assigned theme. Be prepared to share your ideas with the class.

Theme 1 – Culturally Competent Care (Standards 1–3)
Theme 2 – Language Access Services (Standards 4–7)
Theme 3 – Organizational Supports for Cultural Competence (Standards 8–14)

Your Theme Number _____

Strengths	Weaknesses/Challenges	Ideas for Improvement

SESSION 15 Disparities Related to Age

Session Description

This session provides an opportunity for learners to explore the experiences of elderly patients in pursuing health care, and to learn more about special health issues of senior populations and known health and health care disparities. Learners are encouraged to reflect on ways each of them can enhance their patient encounters to help address potential disparities.

Session Objectives

After participation in the session, learners should be better able to:
1. recognize and describe how access, historical, political, environmental, and institutional factors impact health and underlie health and health care disparities for the elderly. (Objective 17 – attitudes, knowledge)
2. identify and discuss key areas of disparities described in *Healthy People 2010* and the Institute of Medicine's Report, *Unequal Treatment*, that relate to the elderly; discuss barriers to eliminating health disparities (Objective 18 – knowledge)
3. describe patterns of health care disparities for the elderly that can result, at least in part, from clinician bias, recognize disparities that are amenable to intervention and value eliminating disparities (Objective 20 – attitudes, knowledge)
4. describe systemic and medical-encounter issues related to health care disparities for the elderly, including communication issues, clinical decision-making, and patient preferences (Objective 21 – knowledge).

Instructional Materials

Flip chart and markers; Death Rates by Race/Ethnicity Table for distribution; video clip – Alicia Mercado from *Worlds Apart* series (*see* Video Resources in Section 7); journal.

Time Schedule

00:00 – 00:05 Session introduction
00:05 – 00:25 Video: Alicia Mercado (13 minutes) and discussion (7 minutes)
00:25 – 00:35 Think-write-share: challenges residents have faced in caring for their elderly patients
00:35 – 00:50 Data review and discussion: elderly health disparities
00:50 – 00:55 Journal
00:55 – 01:00 Session conclusion

Process

1. Session introduction (5 minutes): this session might open by asking the participants if any of them have family stories about the health care challenges of an older person. If no one speaks, the facilitator should have a story prepared from their own family that illustrates challenges in access to and/or quality of care received. Share the session objectives.
2. *Worlds Apart* video and discussion: Alicia Mercado (20 minutes): view the Alicia Mercado documentary together followed by a discussion of barriers to health faced by the patient. These can be elicited from the group and listed on a flip chart. It may be helpful to discuss the role of the physician in this encounter as well, with the group commenting on the degree to which the provider effectively provides culturally responsive care to this patient. They can be reminded of Standards 1–3 of the CLAS Standards from Session 14.
3. Think-write-share (10 minutes): ask the learners to take two minutes to think about and list challenges they have personally faced in caring for elderly patients. They should then take about three minutes to share with a partner. Use the last five minutes or so to elicit comments from the group. Ensure that key concepts are included in the discussion (e.g. health literacy, poly-pharmacy, depression, use of complementary medicine providers, maintaining function/independence, and death/dying).
4. Elderly disparities data (15 minutes): select data regarding health disparities in the elderly from relevant sources (*see* attached list of examples). Distribute and discuss with the group to help them understand the scope of the disparities challenge.

5. Journal (5 minutes): learners are asked to list several barriers to care faced by elderly patients in their own institution. Next, they are asked to list changes in their practice style they hope to adopt to provide better care to geriatric patients.
6. Session conclusion (5 minutes): conclude with a review of the importance of the session's goals and central learning points.

Instructor Notes

Alternatives to showing the Alicia Mercado video include arranging a panel of elderly patients to speak on their health care experiences, or use vignette 6 from the AAFP Quality Care for Diverse Populations video. Another possibility is a group brainstorm on the patient, provider and system contributors to the experience of 'when I cannot be sensitive to my elderly patients'.

Resources

American Academy of Family Physicians. *Quality Care for Diverse Populations*; 2002. Available from: http://www.aafp.org/online/en/home/cme/selfstudy/qualitycarevideo.html

Anderson NB, Bulatao RA, Cohen B, editors. *Critical Perspectives On Racial And Ethnic Differences In Health In Late Life*. Washington DC: National Academies Press; 2004.

Crystal S, Sambamoorthi U, Walkup JT, *et al*. Diagnosis and treatment of depression in the elderly Medicare population: predictors, disparities, and trends. *J Am Geriatr Soc*. 2003 Dec; **51**(12): 1718–28.

Demons JL, Celez R. Geriatrics and End-of-Life Care. In Satcher D, Pamies R. *Multicultural Medicine and Health Disparities*. New York: McGraw Hill; 2006.

Dula, A. The life and death of Miss Mildred: an elderly black woman. *Clin Geriatr Med*. 1994 Aug; **10**(3): 419–30.

Hummer RA, Benjamins MR, Rogers RG. *Racial and Ethnic Disparities in Health and Mortality Among the US Elderly Population* Washington DC: National Academies Press; 2004.

Worlds Apart videos, Fanlight Productions; 2003. Available from: http://www.fanlight.com/home.php

SESSION 15 Disparities Related to Age

Example Health and Health Disparity Information

1. The problem of depression among the elderly became more recognized during the 1990s. The proportion of elderly Medicare patients diagnosed with depression more than doubled from 2.8% in 1992 to 5.8% in 1998, according to a study supported in part by the Agency for Healthcare Research and Quality (HS11825 and HS09566). About two-thirds of those diagnosed with depression received treatment in each year, but those older than 75, those of 'Hispanic or other' ethnicity, and those who did not have supplemental insurance coverage to augment Medicare were significantly less likely to receive treatment. Although blacks were as likely as whites to receive medication or psychotherapy, other racial/ethnic minorities were only half as likely as whites to receive any treatment, controlling for other characteristics. (http://www.ahrq.gov/research/apr04/0404RA5.htm)

2. The poverty rate in 2001 for Hispanic elderly (65 and older) was 22%, which was more than twice the percent for the total older population (10.1%). In 1998, about 2% of Hispanic older persons reported that they had difficulty in obtaining medical care; 5% reported delays in obtaining health care due to cost, and 5% reported that they were unsatisfied with the health care they received. The comparable figures for the total population aged 65 or older were: 2% reported that they had difficulty in obtaining medical care, 4% reported delays in obtaining health care due to cost, and 3% reported that they were unsatisfied with the health care they received.

   A Statistical Profile of Hispanic Older Americans Aged 65+, US Department of Health and Human Services Administration on Aging is available from: http://www.aoa.gov/press/prodsmats/fact/pdf/Facts-on-Hispanic-Elderly092007.pdf

3. In 1999–2002, the percentage of adults who reported using prescription medications in the prior month rose from 36% of those 18–44 years of age to 64% at 45–64 years of age and 85% at 65 years of age and over. In each age group, women were more likely than men to use prescription drugs. In 1999–2002, more than half of adults 65 years of age and over took three or more prescription drugs in the past month.

4. The percentage of adults with three or more chronic conditions increased with age in 2004 from 7% of adults 45–54 years of age to 36% of adults 75 years of age and over. Among adults 45–74 years of age, the percentage of persons reporting three or more chronic conditions rose as income declined. Among adults 75 years of age and over, the percentage of persons with three or more chronic conditions did not vary significantly by income.

5. In 2004, adults 75 years of age and over had a higher rate of visits to the hospital emergency department than other age groups (58 visits per 100 persons compared with 29–45 per 100 persons in other age groups). In 2003–2004, falls accounted for 34% of hospital emergency department injury visits for men 65 years of age and over and 48% for women in that age group. Fall visit rates for adults 85 years and over were almost eight times that of adults 18–64 years of age.

6. Between 1993–1994 and 2003–2004, the hospital discharge rate for cardiac catheterization among adults 75 years of age and over increased 42%, while the rate among adults 65–74 years of age remained stable. By 2003–2004, the cardiac catheterization rate for adults 75 years of age and over had risen to a level similar to that for adults 65–74 years of age.

7. The percentage of the population reporting fair or poor health status, or a limitation of their usual activity due to any chronic condition, increases sharply with age. In 2004, 32% of those 75 years of age and over reported fair or poor health compared with 22% of people age 65–74 and 6% of young adults age 25–44 years.

8. In 2003–2004, about two-thirds of non-Hispanic white older adults and about one-half of Hispanic and non-Hispanic black older adults received influenza vaccinations in the past year.

   Data source for items 3–8: National Center for Health Statistics. *Health, United States, 2006 With Chartbook on Trends in the Health of Americans* Hyattsville, MD: National Center for Health Statistics; 2006. Available from: www.cdc.gov/nchs/data/hus/hus06.pdf

SESSION 16 Building Cultural Skills: the LEARN Mnemonic

Session Description

This session opens with the exercise 'Chicken Soup' to stimulate thinking about culturally congruent care. The learners are then provided with an overview of the LEARN mnemonic (Listen, Explain, Acknowledge, Recommend, Negotiate) and an opportunity to practice negotiation skills with a progressive interview using a trained standardized patient (SP). The session concludes with completion of commitment to change within their journal to further cement new learning in this area.

New in this session: this session introduces the exercise, Chicken Soup, which is described in Section 5.

Session Objectives

After participation in this session, learners should be better able to:
1. describe models of effective cross-cultural communication, assessment, and physician–patient negotiation and identify common challenges in cross-cultural communication (for example, trust, style) (Objective 22 – knowledge)
2. conduct and document a culturally responsive history within the context of family-centered care (Objective 23 – skills)
3. elicit a culture, social, and medical history, including a patient's health beliefs and model of their illness (Objective 23 – skills)
4. demonstrate respect for a patient's culture and health beliefs and use negotiating and problem-solving skills in shared decision-making with a patient (Objective 23 – attitude).

Instructional Materials

Flip chart and markers; didactic presentation on PowerPoint; trained SP; learner journals.

Time Schedule

00:00 – 00:15   Session introduction – Chicken Soup exercise: health beliefs
00:15 – 00:25   Didactic presentation: the LEARN model and negotiation skills
00:25 – 00:45   Progressive interview with SP
00:45 – 00:55   Facilitation of discussion
00:55 – 01:00   Journal and commitment to change

Process

Prior to Session

The SP case should be selected (e.g. Alicia Mercado) or developed and SP trained to be able to answer all questions that might be asked within the context of using the LEARN mnemonic. Try to select a case where health beliefs or cultural lifestyle affect key care decisions, e.g. diabetes, obesity, hypertension (check Section 4 for details on developing an SP case). If you do not have the resources to hire an SP, then you can train a staff member or senior resident to play the role, but the age, gender and ethnicity should match the case as closely as possible.
1. Introduction – Chicken Soup exercise (15 minutes): a number of pieces of flipchart paper are taped to the walls in the classroom. Each participant is given a marker and asked to think back to when they were very young. When someone was sick in their household, what were the family remedies used to help the sick family members to feel better? As they recall these, they are to note them on one of the large sheets of paper on the walls. Next, the facilitator reads some of these aloud, inviting the participants to more fully explain their remedy. It can be interesting to ask them whether they felt the remedy was effective, and whether they would still use it today. The discussion should be upbeat, lively, full of curiosity, and even humor. At the conclusion of the exercise, ask the participants what they take with them as a learning point for the cultural medicine curriculum. It should remind them about the comfort of family remedies and that much of medical treatment happens within the family.

A 'culturally congruent' cure is often very important to people, especially when they are ill. This leads into the discussion about negotiated care.

2. Didactic presentation (10 minutes): during this portion of the session, the instructor reviews the LEARN model of culturally responsive care, and goes on to emphasize the skills of negotiation. Next, the group is asked to suggest what might be required for effective negotiation when Chicken Soup would be appropriate versus when Chicken Soup might not be appropriate (e.g. salt restriction, hypertension).

3. Progressive interview with an SP (20 minutes): the progressive interview uses a time-in/ time-out technique to control the instruction as the learners take turns as the interviewer.

    a) Rules are established in terms of who can call a 'time-out'. Generally, only the current 'interviewer' or the instructor can call a time-out (by making a 'T' with his/her two hands). During a time-out the SP bows his/her head and is 'not in the room'. When 'time-in' is called then the patient returns to the point in the interview where the time-out was called with no apparent interruption in the interview.

    b) Once the interview begins, the interviewer can call time out to ask for advice from the other learners. (Note: let them give the advice – listen more than you talk.) The instructor can also call time out to make a point or to change 'interviewer'.

    c) The interview generally moves fairly quickly, no more than a couple of minutes per learner.

    d) After each learner (or about five learners if the group is large) has had an opportunity to 'interview' the SP, the instructor leads a discussion of the process and the main learning points. Learners may provide feedback to each other as time permits.

4. Facilitation of discussion (10 minutes): over the next 10 minutes the goal is to elicit two to three examples from the group of tough patient care situations where negotiation was needed (whether successfully accomplished or not). The group should be charged with providing suggestions for appropriate data gathering from the patient (e.g. BATHE, Q2, HEADDSS) and for optimal negotiation using LEARN or ETHNIC.

5. Journal and commitment to change (5 minutes): each learner expresses in his/her journal at least one thing they will do differently in their care of patients based on what they learned in this session.

Resources: LEARN, Negotiation

Berlin FA, Fowkes WC Jr. A teaching framework for cross-cultural health care: application in family practice. *West J Med* 1983; **139**: 934–8.

Kagawa-Singer M, Blackhall LJ. Negotiating cross-cultural issues at the end of life: "You got to go where he lives". *JAMA*. 2001 Dec 19; **286**(23): 2993–3001.

Quality Care for Diverse Populations, video with instruction booklet. Kansas City, MO: American Academy of Family Physicians; 2002.

Rosa UW. Impact of cultural competence on medical care: where are we today? *Clin Chest Med*. 2006 Sep; **27**(3): 395–9, v.

Resources: Diabetes, Obesity and Health Beliefs (for SP Case Development)

Albarran NB, Ballesteros MN, Morales GG, *et al.* Dietary behavior and type 2 diabetes care *Patient Educ Couns*. 2006 May; **61**(2): 191–9.

Brown SA, Blozis SA, Kouzekanani K, *et al.* Dosage effects of diabetes self-management education for Mexican Americans: the Starr County Border Health Initiative. *Diabetes Care*. 2005 Mar; **28**(3): 527–32.

Chakraborty BM, Mueller WH, Reeves R, *et al.* For the patient. The importance of health behaviors for better heart health. Migration history, health behaviors, and cardiovascular disease risk factors in overweight Mexican-American women. *Ethn Dis*. 2003; **13**(1): 152.

Clark LT. Issues in minority health: atherosclerosis and coronary heart disease in African Americans. *Med Clin North Am*. 2005 Sep; **89**(5): 977–1001, 994.

Holt P. Challenges and strategies: weight management in type 2 diabetes. *Br J Community Nurs*. 2006 Sep; **11**(9): 376–80.

Melnyk BM, Small L, Morrison-Beedy D, *et al.* Mental health correlates of healthy lifestyle attitudes, beliefs, choices, and behaviors in overweight adolescents. *J Pediatr Health Care*. 2006 Nov–Dec; **20**(6): 401–6.

Resnicow K, Davis R, Rollnick S. Motivational interviewing for pediatric obesity: Conceptual issues and evidence review. *J Am Diet Assoc*. 2006 Dec; **106**(12): 2024–33.

Tan MY. The relationship of health beliefs and complication prevention behaviors of Chinese individuals with Type 2 Diabetes Mellitus. *Diabetes Res Clin Pract*. 2004 Oct; **66**(1): 71–7.

Thornton PL, Kieffer EC, Salabarria-Pena Y, *et al.* Weight, diet, and physical activity-related beliefs and practices among pregnant and postpartum Latino women: the role of social support. *Matern Child Health J*. 2006 Jan; **10**(1): 95–104.

SESSION 17 Integrating Cultural Issues into Case-Based and Literature-Based Sessions (e.g. Mortality-Morbidity, Journal Club, and Conferences on Clinical Topics)

Session Overview

The focus of this session is on encouraging the learners and faculty within a training program to examine how they might incorporate issues related to culture into journal club and mortality-morbidity (quality improvement) conferences, as well as into case-based didactic sessions. The session should open with an activity that engages the learner in thinking about the roles of culture and health disparities in care. The learners are asked to develop a list of all possible questions that might be asked to explore the role of race, ethnicity, culture, class and prior health care disparities on this patient's health status. The group will then review a draft list of questions prepared in advance that might be used in journal club, didactic conferences and mortality-morbidity conferences. The final product of the session will be a tailored list of questions to examine cultural issues within the conferences held in that program.

New in this session: the teaching technique of narrative writing is introduced in this session. You may wish to review the relevant entry in Section 4.

Session Objectives

After participation in the session, learners should be better able to:
1. discuss race, ethnicity, and culture in the context of the medical interview and health care. Show comfort when conversing with patients/colleagues about cultural issues (Objective 9 – attitude, skill)
2. value the importance of curiosity, empathy, and respect in patient care (Objective 11 – attitude)
3. describe the underlying factors and the impact of race/ethnicity, culture, and class on clinical decision-making (Objective 14 – knowledge).

Instructional Materials

Poster board (large Post-a-Note pad often works best); copy of the CC curriculum and draft list of CC questions that could be used in a) M&M (quality improvement) conference, b) journal club, and c) didactic sessions focused on specific topics or medical problems.

Time Schedule

00:00 – 00:05 Session introduction
00:05 – 00:15 Narrative exercise, think-pair-share
00:15 – 00:25 Debriefing
00:25 – 00:50 Review of draft questions and discussion
00:50 – 00:55 Concluding activities
00:55 – 01:00 Journal

Process

1. Introduction (5 minutes): the session introduction provides an overview of the session and describes how it is part of the larger culturally responsive care curriculum.
2. Narrative writing from the patient's point of view and think-pair-share (10 minutes): tell the participants that they will have five minutes to complete a brief narrative from the point of view of a patient and will then have five minutes to share their narrative with a partner. Encourage the learners to share only what they are comfortable sharing during the think-pair-share.

   Case scenario: Mrs Williams is your patient. Your team has decided that the best treatment for her disease requires that she be placed on an experimental protocol. Mrs Williams is an African-American woman who grew up in the south and does not trust the health care system.

Directions: Write in her voice, what 'you' as the patient would like to know about the study as you consider this option? Then share as much of your narrative as you are comfortable sharing, with your assigned/selected partner. Then, as a pair combine your lists of questions into a single list.

3. Debriefing (10 minutes): ask for a volunteer to share their list – record the items on a blank flip chart sheet. Ask the group to expand on the list based on what they wrote and note common items. Be sure to discuss the importance of the trust relationship in gaining informed consent for necessary treatment, as well as in gaining initial information needed to make diagnoses and provided excellent care.
4. Review of questions for conferences (25 minutes): pass out the lists of questions provided. Begin the discussion with the journal club list. Do the topical list last as it was not part of their narrative activity. Get as far as you can with the lists, but be sure to leave 10 minutes at the end for the closing activities and the journal.
5. Closing activities (5 minutes): 1. discuss with the group the feasibility of incorporating these questions into their regular conferences. Ask them for the best way to ensure that these issues are included. 2. conclude with a review of the importance of the session's goals and central learning points, inviting learners to take the session contents directly back into their clinical work.
6. Journal (5 minutes): learners have the opportunity to write about any new learning based on the narrative activity or on the discussion.

Resources

Anderson LM, Scrimshaw SC, Fullilove MT, *et al*. Task Force on Community Preventive Services. Culturally competent healthcare systems: A systematic review. *Am J Prev Med*. 2003 Apr; **24**(3 Suppl.): 68–79.

Crandall SJ, George G, Marion GS, *et al*. Applying theory to the design of cultural competency training for medical students: a case study. *Acad Med*. 2003 Jun; **78**(6): 588–94.

Kohn, LT, Corrigan, JM and Donaldson, MS. To Err is Human: Building a Safer Health System. (IOM Report). Washington DC: National Academies Press; 2000.

Kripalani S, Bussey-Jones J, Katz MG, *et al*. A prescription for cultural competence in medical education. *J Gen Intern Med*. 2006 Oct; **21**(10): 1116–20.

Schulman KA, Berlin JA, Harless W, *et al*. The effect of race and sex on physicians' recommendations for cardiac catheterization. *N Engl J Med*. 1999; **340**: 618–26.

Potential Conference Questions by Cultural Competence Curriculum Objective

Questions Related to Research Articles and Presentations of Literature

#	Objectives	Literature-Related Questions
3	Value the importance of diversity in health care and address the challenges and opportunities it poses. (A)	Who were the participants in the study? How were they selected? How well did they reflect the diversity of our patient population?
7	Describe historical models of common health beliefs (for example, illness in the context of 'hot and cold'), and identify questions about health practices and beliefs that might be important in a specific local community. (K)	How were the health beliefs and cultural context of patients taken into consideration in this study? What more could have been done?
19	Identify and discuss key areas of disparities described in *Healthy People 2010* and the Institute of Medicine's Report *Unequal Treatment* and discuss barriers to eliminating health disparities. (K)	Was the issue of health care disparities addressed in the article? Should it have been? Why or why not?
26	Critically appraise the literature as it relates to health disparities, including systems issues and quality in health care. (Sk)	How will the results of the study impact health care disparities – improve, make worse, no impact? Why?

Questions Related to Specific Patient Cases (Mortality-Morbidity Conference, etc.)

#	Objectives	Conference Questions
8	Identify healing traditions and beliefs of patients and/or their families, including ethno-medical beliefs. Ask questions in a non-judgmental manner to elicit patient preferences, listen and respond appropriately to patient feedback about key cross-cultural issues. Elicit additional information about ethno-medical conditions and ethno-medical healers. (A, K, Sk)	Any role for alternative or complementary medicine for this patient? Could it help or have helped? Did it hinder?
12	Recognize their own potential for bias and stereotyping, be able to identify their own stereotypes and biases and explore how their attitudes, biases and stereotypes affect clinical encounters, clinical decision-making and quality of care. (A, K)	Have the attitudes, biases or stereotypes of providers (related to race, ethnicity, class, economic status, sex, sexual preference, religion, culture, etc.) affected care and/or outcomes for this patient? If yes, how?
15	Describe strategies for reducing physician's own biases, and those of others, and demonstrate strategies to assess, manage, and reduce bias and its effects in the clinical encounter and in clinical practice. (Sk)	How can we reduce the impact of any biases in the care of future patients?
17	Recognize and describe how access, historical, political, environmental, and institutional factors (including racism and discrimination) impact health and underlie health and health care disparities. (A, K)	Were any health care disparities already affecting the patient's health status prior to us seeing the patient? How can we avoid health disparities for future patients?
18	Identify how race, ethnicity and social determinants of health (e.g., education, culture, socioeconomic status, housing and employment) affect health and health care quality, cost, and outcomes. (K)	Any concerns about the patient's ability or willingness to adhere to the treatment plan, and how did this play a role in outcomes?
20	Describe patterns of health care disparities that can result, at least in part, from clinician bias. Recognize disparities that are amenable to intervention and value eliminating disparities. (A, K)	What action can we take to help eliminate any disparity affecting this patient?

cont.

#	Objectives	Conference Questions
21	Describe systemic and medical-encounter issues related to health care disparities, including communication issues, clinical decision-making, and patient preferences. (K)	Any discrepancies between the assessment and plan, and the patient's health belief system? Anything omitted from the plan based on 'who' this patient is (e.g. likeable, deserving, living circumstances, etc) or based on patient preferences? Consequences?
22	Describe models of effective cross-cultural communication, assessment, and physician-patient negotiation and identify common challenges in cross-cultural communication (for example, trust, style). (K)	Were there communication challenges in the care of this patient? If so, how were they addressed and what was the impact on care and outcomes?
25	Assess and enhance patient adherence based on the patient's explanatory model. Describe ways to enhance patient adherence by collaborating with traditional and other community healers. (K, Sk)	If patient adherence was an issue, what might we do to enhance it?

Questions Related to Topical Presentations

#	Objectives	Topic-Related Questions
4	Identify patterns of national data on health, health care disparities, and quality of health care, and be able to describe it in a worldwide immigration context. (K)	What patterns of disparities have been identified in relation to this topic/medical problem?
5	Discuss the epidemiology of health and health care disparities for the local community using *Healthy People 2010* and other resources. (K, Sk)	Related to this topic/medical problem, what health care disparities exist locally, in the county, state or nation? How are we doing in addressing them for our patients?
6	Value the importance of social determinants and community factors on health and strive to address them. (A, Sk)	In relation to the topic/medical problem, are there social determinants in our community that contribute to disparities and how can we address them?
7	Describe historical models of common health beliefs (for example, illness in the context of 'hot and cold'), and identify questions about health practices and beliefs that might be important in a specific local community. (K)	Are there any common health beliefs or practices in our community related to this topic/medical problem? How should we address them?
8	Identify healing traditions and beliefs of patients and/or their families, including ethno-medical beliefs. Ask questions in a non-judgmental manner to elicit patient preferences, listen and respond appropriately to patient feedback about key cross-cultural issues. Elicit additional information about ethno-medical conditions and ethno-medical healers. (A, K, Sk)	What role do alternative or ethno-medical healers play in our community in relation to this topic/medical problem? How should we be addressing this in our care plans?

SESSION 18 Focused Review of Local, State, and National Health Data

(Infant Mortality and Natality Indicators)

Session Description

This annual session (sessions 8, 18 and 28) is designed to provide the opportunity for learners to review actual health status data: national, state and particularly local. In the state of California, data is provided annually that compares each county with all other counties, with the state average, and with the *Healthy People 2010* goal for a variety of health issues. This data should be reviewed (check you own state Department of Health for similar data) along with any data collected in relation to PBLI (practice-based learning and improvement) goals for your program's clinic or hospital. Learners may also be able to look at the data on their own patient population in relation to program goals or *Healthy People 2010* goals. *Healthy People 2010* is a very extensive document addressing a wide variety of issues. Familiarity with both it and the *Healthy People Midcourse Review* will increase understanding of the goals and the progress from 2000 to 2005. Since this is an annual session, the program has the opportunity to select different areas of emphasis each year, providing a variety of foci for learner review.

Session Objectives

After participation in the session, learners should be better able to:
1. identify patterns of national data on health, health care disparities, and quality of health care, and describe them in a worldwide immigration context (Objective 4 – knowledge)
2. discuss the epidemiology of health and health care disparities for the local community using *Healthy People 2010* and other resources (Objective 5 – knowledge, skill)
3. critically appraise the literature as it relates to health disparities, including systems issues and quality in health care (Objective 26 – skill).

Instructional Materials

National, regional and *Healthy People 2010* data (copies made for each person or each small group); local hospital, clinic, and individual resident data if available; small group assignments for this session based on the data focus selected.

Time Schedule

00:00 – 00:05 Session introduction
00:05 – 00:30 Small group data review
00:30 – 00:50 Facilitation of group discussion of common themes
00:50 – 01:00 Conclusion of session, journal or commitment to change

Process

Prior to Session

   a) Select the topic for data review from those included in *Healthy People 2010*. Select a topic that resonates with the local community. Below are several suggestions – our suggestion for Session 18 is infant mortality.
   b) Plan a relevant small group assignment that requires the students/residents to review the data in a meaningful manner (generally a series of questions to answer, *see* Session 8 for a sample assignment).
1. Introduction (5 minutes): this session should begin with an opener that draws the learners' attention to the focus of the session. A quote or a statistic could open the session, or the learners could be presented with a challenge in relation to health care within the clinic, health center or community where data would be important in addressing an issue.
2. Small group exercises – data review (25 minutes): provide the pre-planned assignment to each group along with the data sheets prepared in advance. Monitor the progress of the groups and provide assistance in examining the data if required.

3. Debriefing of exercise and discussion of challenges and common themes (20 minutes): use facilitation to debrief the exercise. Be careful to include all groups in reporting the answers to the questions in your pre-planned exercise. For each question, ask a different group to provide their answer first. Ask all groups for any other additional or differing interpretations and ideas. Encourage the students to discuss any disagreements. Return to the data if necessary.

4. Session conclusion and journal (10 minutes): learners should be asked how they might make use of data in their own practices. Ask them to commit to making just one change over the next year in relation to use of data to enhance their evidence-based practice.

Data Sources

Agency for Health Care Quality and Research: http://www.ahrq.gov/qual/measurix.htm
On this website, you will find two reports: 1. the annual National Healthcare Disparities Reports (NHDR) examining the distribution of improvement in health care quality; and 2. the National Healthcare Quality Report (NHQR), addressing the current state of health care quality.

California Center for Health Statistics: http://www.dhs.ca.gov/hisp/chs/OHIR/reports/
The site provides a wide variety of data reports related to the health status of Californians. Of particular interest are the annual County Health Status Profiles that provide comparative data for all California counties in relation to each other and to the *Healthy People 2010* goals. Other data include deaths by zip code, and statistics for many disease states and causes of death.

Centers for Disease Control Office of Minority Health: http://www.cdc.gov/omh/AboutUs/disparities.htm
Obtain data on health disparities at the Center for Disease Control.

DHHS Office of Minority Health Resource Center: http://www.omhrc.gov/
This site has information in three categories: staying healthy, health disparities, and communities in action.

Healthy People 2010: http://www.healthypeople.gov/Document/tableofcontents.htm
Healthy People 2010 provides a large set of health objectives for the nation to achieve by the year 2010. The *Healthy People Midcourse Review* reports progress toward meeting the *Healthy People 2010* goals http://www.healthypeople.gov/data/midcourse/default.htm#pubs

Kaiser Family Foundation – State Health Facts: http://www.statehealthfacts.org/cgi-bin/healthfacts.cgi
This site provides free, up-to-date, and easy-to-use health data on over 500 health topics for all 50 states.

National Center for Health Statistics: www.cdc.gov/nchs/data/hus/hus06.pdf
Health, United States 2006, with Chartbook on Trends in the Health of Americans provides data for the US in comparison to other nations and a wide variety of health data and comparisons including those by race, ethnicity, gender, and age. Downloads as a PDF document.

SESSIONS 8, 18 AND 28 Focused Review of Local, State, and National Health Data

Selecting Topics for Data Review

Potential Topics

1. Leading causes of death (http://www.cdc.gov/nchs/fastats/deaths.htm)
   Number of deaths for leading causes of death in the United States in 2005:
   - Heart disease: 652,091
   - Cancer: 559,312
   - Stroke (cerebrovascular diseases): 143,579
   - Chronic lower respiratory diseases: 130,933
   - Accidents (unintentional injuries): 117,809
   - Diabetes: 75,119
   - Alzheimer's disease: 71,599
   - Influenza/pneumonia: 63,001
   - Nephritis, nephrotic syndrome, and nephrosis: 43,901
   - Septicemia: 34,136
2. Topics within *Healthy People 2010*: access and medical topics: http://www.healthypeople.gov/Document/tableofcontents.htm
3. Leading health indicators – *Healthy People 2010* tracks a group of leading health indicators that include: physical activity, overweight and obesity, tobacco use, substance abuse, responsible sexual behavior, mental health, injury and violence, environmental quality, and immunization. The leading health indicators were selected on the basis of their 'ability to motivate action, the availability of data to measure progress, and their importance as public health issues'. http://www.healthypeople.gov/LHI/lhiwhat.htm
4. Access to health care areas reported in state level reports. In the annual California County Health Status Profiles, mortality statistics are provided in the following areas: all causes of death, motor vehicle crashes, unintentional injuries, firearm injuries, homicide, suicide, all cancer deaths, lung cancer, female breast cancer, coronary heart disease, cerebrovascular disease (stroke), drug-induced deaths, and diabetes. http://www.dhs.ca.gov/hisp/chs/OHIR/reports/healthstatusprofiles/default.htm
5. The three areas we are suggesting are: 1. injuries and violence (a leading health indicator); 2. infant mortality and early pregnancy care; 3. diseases from among those where both state and national data are available (could have one for each small group among those most prevalent in your community).

SESSION 18 Focused Review of Local, State, and National Health Data

Sample Data Sources for Infant Mortality and Natality Indicators

1. 2007 County Health Status Profiles for the state of California. http://www.dhs.ca.gov/hisp/chs/OHIR/reports/healthstatusprofiles/default.htm
   a) Birth cohort infant mortality under one year of age per 1000 live births (24A – 24E)
      24A. All race/ethnic groups infant mortality (pages 49–50)
      24B. Asian/pacific islander race group infant mortality (pages 51–52)
      24C. Black race group infant mortality (pages 53–54)
      24D. Hispanic ethnic group infant mortality (pages 55–56)
      24E. White race group infant mortality (pages 57–58)
   b) Natality indicators per 100 live births or 1000 population (25 – 27B)
      25. Low birthweight infants (pages 59–60)
      26. Births to adolescent mothers, 15–19 years old per 1000 live births (pages 61–62)
      27A. Prenatal care not begun during the first trimester (pages 63–64)
      27B. Adequate/adequate plus prenatal care (APNCU Index) (pages 65–66)
   c) Breastfeeding initiation rates per 100 live births
      28. Breastfeeding initiation during early post partum (pages 67–68)
2. National Center for Health Statistics. *Health, United States, 2006 With Chartbook on Trends in the Health of Americans*. www.cdc.gov/nchs/data/hus/hus06.pdf Sections on Fertility and Natality (Tables 4–18), Infant Mortality (Tables 19–25)
3. In California, *Healthy People 2010* Objectives Focus Area 16: Maternal, Infant and Child Health. http://www.dhs.ca.gov/chs/OHIR/hp2010/hc2010progress.htm
4. *National Healthcare Quality Report*, 2006. http://www.ahrq.gov/qual/measurix.htm. Section on Maternal and Child Health, pages 52–58
5. *National Healthcare Disparities Report*, 2006. http://www.ahrq.gov/qual/measurix.htm. Sections on Women (pages 158–164) and children (pages 165–76)

SESSION 18 Focused Review of Local, State, and National Health Data

Infant Mortality and Natality Indicators

Sample Small Group Assignment

Directions. Infant mortality is one indicator of the health of our patient population and of the health of the nation. As part of your Practice-Based Learning and Improvement, you will want to track these statistics for your patient population. However, in order to understand what your data means you need comparison data.

1. According to the 2007 infant mortality County Health Status Profiles for the State of California, a) how well is Los Angeles county doing in relation to other counties, b) in comparison to Healthy People 2010 goals, and c) between the various ethnic groups listed?

2. Look further in the National Center for Health Statistics, *Health, United States, 2007 with Chartbook on Trends in the Health of Americans* for the areas of Prenatal Care (Table 7, page 138), Early Pre-Natal Care by race and Hispanic origin (Table 8, pages 139–141), infant mortality (Table 19, pages 159–161) and neonatal mortality (Table 24, pages 169–171). What are the differences, if any, by ethnicity/race among the groups nationally? In California? If available, how does our local data compare?

3. Take a look at some other data sources:
   a) National Healthcare Quality Report, 2006, Section on Maternal and Child health, for California. http://www.ahrq.gov/qual/measurix.htm
   b) National Healthcare Disparities Report, 2006, Section on children. http://www.ahrq.gov/qual/measurix.htm
   c) Healthy California 2010, Focus Area 16, Maternal, Infant and Child health

How is State of California doing in relation to the indicators used in relation to Maternal, Infant and Child health? Where do we excel? What needs more work?

SESSION 19 Annual Second Year Resident Patient Case Presentations: Cultural Issues in Negotiated Care

Session Description

This annual session (sessions 9, 19 and 29) is an application and integration exercise for second year residents to use the materials learned in the cultural competence curriculum up to this point. (With other learners this activity would be non-repeating and occur at the end of Unit V.) The expanded case format is used, with relevant cultural issues discussed. Each presenter will have prepared a brief description of a patient case where the patient's health beliefs were an issue in negotiating a care plan. The learner should demonstrate knowledge of the patient, and of any relevant historical model of health beliefs. Learners should be encouraged to include cases where alternative or ethno-medical healers were incorporated. Approximately five to seven learners can share within a one-hour session. Small groups with faculty group leaders can be used to allow more learners to present within a single session.

Session Objectives

After participation in the session, learners should be better able to:
1. describe historical models of common health beliefs (for example, illness in the context of 'hot and cold'), and identify questions about health practices and beliefs that might be important in a specific local community (Objective 7 – knowledge)
2. identify healing traditions and beliefs of patients and/or their families, including ethno-medical beliefs and describe (Objective 8 – skill)
3. describe models of effective cross-cultural communication, assessment, and physician–patient negotiation and identify common challenges in cross-cultural communication (for example, trust, style) (Objective 22 – knowledge)
4. assess and enhance patient adherence based on the patient's explanatory model. Describe ways to enhance patient adherence by collaborating with traditional and other community healers (Objective 25 – knowledge, skill).

Instructional Materials

Presentation assignment and guidelines, distributed some weeks prior to the presentation date to learners who will be presenting cases; materials requested by residents/students to facilitate case presentations; session objectives; journals.

Time Schedule

00:00 – 00:03 Session introduction
00:03 – 00:45 Case presentations (maximum of seven six-minute case presentations)
00:45 – 00:55 Group discussion of common themes and session conclusion
00:55 – 01:00 Journal and commitment to change

Process

Distribute presentation assignment and guidelines (attached) some weeks prior to the presentation date to learners who have been assigned to present cases. Instructors may want to review proposed cases with learners prior to the presentation date for appropriateness and relevance.
1. Introduction (3 minutes): this session requires only a brief introduction to present the session objectives to the learners, and explain how this session is part of the larger culturally responsive care curriculum.
2. Case presentations (42 minutes): each learner presents a case example of their work with a patient that illustrates culturally responsive care in terms of negotiating a culturally responsive treatment plan, incorporation of patient's health beliefs in treatment plan, as well as collaboration with alternative or ethno-medical healers. Relevant health outcomes should be mentioned.

3. Group discussion of common themes and session conclusion (10 minutes): use facilitation to engage all learners in discussion. Invite learners to identify any commonalities they observed in the case presentations in terms of clinical challenges and positive interventions.
4. Journal (5 minutes): learners have the opportunity to write about their new learning based on the case presentations (both from preparing their own as well as listening to others). Encourage learners to commit to take one lesson directly back into their work.

Cautionary Note

Once learners begin this project, they will be challenged to keep their presentation brief and focused on the cultural aspects of the case. They may require guidance in pulling together relevant data instead of potentially presenting typical history and physical data, which may not be relevant to the task at hand.

Instructor Note

This exercise could easily be expanded into 30 minutes per learner, if time permits in your curriculum. Each learner presentation would be 20 minutes with 10 minutes for discussion. The presentation outline might be as follows: 1. case presentation; 2. formal discussion of the health belief system held by the patient; 3. a brief description of the cross-cultural communication model used by the resident; and 4. personal insights gained by the resident in the exploration of the case. Learners might use a PowerPoint presentation format to share their information with the group. Each presentation would be followed by discussion. The other learners should complete a formal evaluation of each of these presentations to assist the presenter in honing presentation skills.

Resources

Aberegg SK, Terry PB. Medical decision-making and healthcare disparities: the physician's role. *J Lab Clin Med*. 2004 Jul; **144**(1): 11–7.

Balsa AI, Seiler N, McGuire TG, *et al*. Clinical uncertainty and healthcare disparities. *Am J Law Med*. 2003; **29**(2–3): 203–19.

Lewis-Fernandez R, Diaz, N. The cultural formulation: a method for assessing cultural factors affecting the clinical encounter. *Psychiatr Quart*. 2002; **73**(4): 271–95.

Lu FG, Lim R, Mezzich JE. Issues in the assessment and diagnosis of culturally diverse individuals. In Oldham J, Riba M, editors. *Review of Psychiatry*, Vol. 14. Washington DC: American Psychiatric Press; 1995. pp. 477–510.

Thiel de Bocanegra H, Gany F. Good provider, good patient: changing behaviors to eliminate disparities in healthcare. *Am J Manag Care*. 2004 Sep; **10** Spec No: SP20–8.

SESSION 19 – RESIDENT HANDOUT Cultural Medicine Case Presentation Preparation Guidelines

You are to prepare a six-minute presentation of a case that illustrates your culturally responsive work with a patient. The presentation will be on (insert date here), and you will be one of (insert number) presenters that day.

Objectives
The objectives of these presentations are to:
1. describe the patient's historical model of health belief (if applicable) and the questions about health practices and beliefs that were important to your understanding of that patient's model
2. identify healing traditions and beliefs of your patient and/or their family, including ethno-medical beliefs and use of ethno-medical healers
3. describe any model of cross-cultural communication, assessment, and provider–patient negotiation that you used and identify any challenges you faced (for example: trust, style)
4. if appropriate, describe how you worked to enhance patient adherence by collaborating with traditional and other community healers.

Instructions
1. Select a case where a health belief of the patient was relevant to your care. You should be able to discuss the health belief in the context of any relevant historical model of health care belief. In selecting your case pick one where negotiation of a care plan that incorporated the patient's health beliefs was important and/or where collaboration with alternative or ethno-medical healers took place.
2. You may discuss your case selection with the course instructor in terms of appropriateness and relevance of the case to the cultural medicine curriculum and session goals.
3. Given the brief time allotted for the presentation, be very judicious in selecting which aspects of the case to include. For example, share only case history data that directly applies to the health belief in question, use of alternative/complementary medicine and any cultural negotiation of the treatment plan.
4. Be sure to share insights you have gained about the health belief in question from research you did on that belief.
5. Practice your presentation – six minutes is brief, timing is important.

SESSION 20 Annual Review of Individual Cultural Competency Commitments

Session Description

The final session in each year of the three-year curriculum (sessions 10, 20 and 30) provides an opportunity for each learner to use reflection and self-assessment to reflect upon their journal entries and their progress to date. Learners will be provided the opportunity to share with each other, if they chose to, some of their areas of positive growth, as well as remaining challenges. There will also be time for general discussion in relation to ways for reducing bias of the providers and for addressing disparities for patients within their practice environment. The group might select one thing to work on over the next academic year. In the second and third year, the group should spend some time in this session discussing progress over the past year on their target goal.

Session Objectives

After participation in the session, learners should be better able to:

1. become aware of their own cultural heritage, gender, class, ethnic-racial identity, sexual orientation, disability, age, and spirituality; be able to reflect on it and describe it (Objective 2 – awareness, skill)
2. recognize their own potential for bias and stereotyping, be able to identify their own stereotypes and biases and explore how their attitudes, biases and stereotypes affect clinical encounters, clinical decision-making and quality of care (Objective 12 – awareness, knowledge)
3. describe strategies for reducing physician's own biases, and those of others and demonstrate strategies to assess, manage, and reduce bias and its effects in the clinical encounter and in clinical practice (Objective 15 – skill)
4. describe patterns of health care disparities that can result, at least in part, from clinician bias, recognize disparities that are amenable to intervention and value eliminating disparities (Objective 20 – attitude, knowledge).

Instructional Materials

Flip chart and pens; the entire set of objectives for the cultural competence curriculum for review; collected learner materials for each learner (presentations, quizzes, reflective writings, journals, etc.) should be distributed to each learner at the start of the session.

Time Schedule

00:00 – 00:05   Session introduction
00:05 – 00:20   Independent review of journal, reflections and commitments
00:20 – 00:40   Open discussion
00:40 – 00:55   Plan for change/think-pair-share
00:55 – 01:00   Session conclusion

Process

1. Introduction (5 minutes): this session requires only a brief introduction to the importance of this session as part of the larger culturally responsive care curriculum.
2. Independent review (15 minutes): learners are provided with their complete collection of materials gathered over the course of their participation in the cultural medicine curriculum (including their journals and any orientation materials for first year residents). Ask them to review the materials with an eye to their positive growth, areas for further and future growth, the degree to which they have been able to fulfill their commitments, and any barriers faced in fulfilling those commitments. Learners may wish to highlight outstanding learning experiences and/or clinical encounters over the past year.
3. Open discussion (20 minutes): here the group is invited to share their findings from the independent review. Successes, frustrations, and barriers can be highlighted by the group facilitator on flip charts at the front of the room. A revisiting of the cultural curriculum

objectives can be helpful and included as part of this discussion. The skills of facilitation will help ensure a student-centered discussion.

4. Plan for change/think-write-share (15 minutes): looking to the future, learners are asked to write their personal goals for professional growth toward culturally responsive care, including any personal areas of bias, stereotyping and/or discomfort. Next, each learner shares these with a partner, and finally the group as a whole joins a larger discussion of future learning goals.

5. Session conclusion (5 minutes): this is an opportunity to thank the learners for their input today and over this segment of the curriculum (Sessions A, B, C and 11–20) and remind them that the curriculum uses a spiral model. In the next year, the learners will revisit each of the six units in the third year of the curriculum (Sessions 21–30).

Instructor Note

Learners often have a tendency to focus more on the negative than the positive in their own professional trajectory. It is important that the facilitator help learners share both frustrations and observed areas of growth and accomplishment in a balanced fashion.

Resources

Betancourt JR. Cultural competence and medical education: many names, many perspectives, one goal. *Acad Med*. 2006 Jun; **81**(6): 499–501.

Chambers N. Close encounters: the use of critical reflective analysis as an evaluation tool in teaching and learning. *J Adv Nurs*. 1999; **29**(4): 950–7.

Like RC. Culturally competent family medicine: transforming clinical practice and ourselves. *Am Fam Physician*. 2005 Dec; **72**(11): 2189.

Murray-Garcia JL, Harrell S, Garcia JA, *et al*. Self-reflection in multicultural training: be careful what you ask for. *Acad Med*. 2005 Jul; **80**(7): 694–701.

SESSION 21 Power, Privilege, and the Patient Encounter

Session Description

This session explores the concepts of power, privilege, and the patient encounter through the viewing of a video clip entitled *Sickle Cell in the ER* and a narrative writing exercise that develops out of the video material. The video depicts a number of ways in which patient disempowerment can contribute to health care disparities. The group is asked to reflect on how power dynamics can play out in the doctor–patient encounter.

This session opens the third year of the curriculum. If your program has not instituted the use of learner portfolios, we recommend that you begin to do so this year. Learners will have a variety of items to place in a portfolio that will demonstrate the ongoing impact of the curriculum, including narrative/reflective writings, student presentations, and commitments to change.

New in this session: this session introduces the teaching methods, best-worst warm-up and portfolio, described in Section 4.

Session Objectives

After participation in the session, learners should be better able to:
1. recognize their own potential for bias and stereotyping, be able to identify their own stereotypes and biases and explore how their attitudes, biases and stereotypes affect clinical encounters, clinical decision-making and quality of care (Objective 12 – attitudes)
2. describe strategies for reducing physician's own biases, and those of others, and demonstrate strategies to assess, manage, and reduce bias and its effects in the clinical encounter and in clinical practice (Objective 15 – skill, knowledge)
3. describe the inherent power imbalance between physician and patient and how it affects the clinical encounter (Objective 16 – knowledge).

Instructional Materials

Video clip: *Sickle Cell in the ER* is a 5-minute video scenario included in *Cultural Issues in the Clinical Setting*, Kaiser Permanente, 2002 – Series A (*see* Video and DVD Resources, Section 7); VCR and monitor; flip chart and markers; a notebook for each learner to use to build his/her portfolio.

Time Schedule

00:00 – 00:05	Session opener
00:05 – 00:10	Video clip: *Sickle Cell in the ER*
00:10 – 00:15	Narrative writing exercise (placed in portfolio)
00:15 – 00:30	Discussion and sharing of writing
00:30 – 00:40	Best-worst warm-up
00:40 – 00:50	Group discussion: potential power violations in doctor/patient encounters
00:50 – 01:00	Portfolio and commitment to change

Process

1. Session introduction (5 minutes): suggested introduction – a quote from Jimi Hendrix:

   'When the power of love overcomes the love of power, the world will know peace.' On your flip chart make a line down the middle. At the top of one side write 'The Power of Love' and on the other side write 'The Love of Power'. Ask the learners how these two concepts, in practice, can contribute positively or negatively to the doctor–patient relationship and/ or to other relationships in the health care team? Write all ideas, with minimal discussion. This is a tease – an opener – to grab their attention. When the ideas stop coming, move on to the video.

2. Video clip – *Sickle Cell in the ER* (5 minutes): this video vignette portrays a situation in which a young African-American male does not receive needed care, due to an unrecognized bias in how he is treated in the waiting room.

3. Narrative writing (5 minutes): participants are asked to choose any of the characters in the video clip, including another patient in the waiting room who witnesses the events. This is a point-of-view narrative so the learner writes the perspective of the individual they have chosen. Instruct them thus 'Write in the voice of the person you choose, representing his/her thoughts, impressions and reactions to what happened. You may use poetry or prose.'

4. Think-write-share and discussion of narratives (15 minutes): ask the learners to partner with someone and share their narrative (approximately 5 minutes). There are several ways to proceed with the sharing of writing. Perhaps, as in the think-write-share technique, learners read their narrative in pairs or small groups, then later volunteers can share with the group as a whole. If the group knows each other well, then volunteers are invited to read their narratives to the group as a whole. Allow for a brief discussion of any remaining reflections or questions that arose from the video scenario.

5. Best-worst warm-up (10 minutes): ask the group to call out the benefits and potential abuses/problems of the physician unavoidably holding more power in the doctor–patient relationship

6. Group discussion (10 minutes): potential power violations in the doctor–patient relationship. This discussion may begin with an open question about the definition of power, and the dynamics of power in the doctor–patient relationship. Perhaps learners have examples of when, as patients, they felt disempowered or empowered by the physician. Solicit examples of power abuse, perhaps opening discussion about the Tuskegee experiments.

7. Portfolio and commitment to change (10 minutes): distribute the notebooks and if necessary, introduce the learners to the concept of a cultural competence portfolio. The portfolio should have dividers for all sessions (21–30) where learners will be adding materials. Ask the learners to complete a commitment to change form and add it along with their narrative writing product to the portfolio.

Cautionary Note

Discussions of power and privilege can grow quite emotional given the history of power abuses in this country, and perhaps in the lives of participants. It is important that the instructor be comfortable with frank discussions of power dynamics in a group setting.

Resources

Byrd WM, Clayton L. *An American Health Dilemma: A medical history of African Americans and the problem of race: Beginnings to 1900.* New York: Routledge; 2000.

Byrd WM, Clayton L. *An American Health Dilemma: Race, medicine and health care in the United States 1900–2000.* New York: Routledge; 2002.

Goodyear-Smith F, Buetow S. Power issues in the doctor-patient relationship. *Health Care Anal.* 2001; **9**(4): 449–62.

Pinderhughes E. *Understanding Race, Ethnicity and Power.* New York: The Free Press; 1989.

SESSION 22 Medical Interpretation: Use of a Live Interpreter

Session Description

This very important session introduces learners to the skills necessary to provide medical care across linguistic barriers. The session begins with a review of the CLAS Standards referring to linguistically sensitive care. This is followed by the viewing of an instructional video by the Cross Cultural Health Program, entitled *Communicating Effectively through an Interpreter* (*see* Video/DVD Resources in Section 7).

Session Objectives

After participation in this session, learners should be better able to:
1. recognize and describe institutional cultural issues for own institution and discuss the CLAS Standards (Objective 10 – knowledge)
2. demonstrate respect for a patient's cultural and health beliefs and use negotiating and problem-solving skills in shared decision-making with a patient (Objective 23 – attitude, skills)
3. describe the functions of an interpreter and effective ways of working with an interpreter. Identify when an interpreter is needed and collaborate effectively with an interpreter (Objective 24 – knowledge, skills).

Instructional Materials

Text of CLAS Standards 4–7 for distribution; videotape: *Communicating Effectively through an Interpreter*; handout: how to access language services at your clinical facilities (to be prepared at your institution).

Time Schedule

00:00 – 00:05 Session introduction
00:05 – 00:10 Didactic presentation: review of CLAS Standards 4–7
00:10 – 00:40 Video: *Communicating Effectively through an Interpreter*
00:40 – 00:50 Think-pair-share and debriefing
00:50 – 01:00 Session conclusion and commitment to change

Process

1. Session introduction (5 minutes): the introduction for this session should be very brief and grab the learners' attention. For many learners this is not seen as an exciting topic. Look for an opener (quote, brief story from your own practice, cartoon, etc.) that will help the learners appreciate the importance of the topic.
2. Didactic presentation (5 minutes): the instructor distributes the CLAS Standards 4–7 and reviews these with the learners, emphasizing the importance and challenges of providing excellent care in the face of language barriers.
3. View the video (30 minutes): prior to class, preview the video and select one or two stopping points to check learners' understanding of concepts and entertain questions. Instruct the learners to make notes of the most important points as they watch. Monitor the learners as they view the video *Communicating Effectively through an Interpreter* and pause it for discussion one (or more) times based on audience need and the points that you pre-selected as stop points.
4. Think-pair-share (10 minutes): allow the learners to discuss what they noted from the video using the think-pair-share technique, and then conduct a short debriefing of the video with the entire group. This is also a good opportunity to answer any questions the video may have raised for the learners in relation to live and/or telephonic interpretation. Learners should be instructed in how to access language services at their clinical sites and those instructions should be distributed at this point.
5. Session conclusion (10 minutes): conclude with a review of the importance of the session's goals and central learning points, have them record their commitment to change and encourage the learners to take their commitments directly back into their clinical work.

Resources

Ahmed R, Bowen J, O'Donnell W. Cultural competence and language interpreter services in Minnesota: results of a needs assessment survey administered to physician members of the Minnesota Medical Association. *Minnesota Med*. 2004 Dec; **87**(12): 40–2.

Anderson LM, Scrimshaw SC, Fullilove MT, *et al*. Task Force on Community Preventive Services. Culturally competent healthcare systems: a systematic review. *Am J Prevent Med*. 2003 Apr; **24**(3 Suppl.): 68–79.

Betancourt JR, Green AR, Carrillo JE, *et al*. Defining cultural competence: a practical framework for addressing racial/ethnic disparities in health and health care. *Public Health Reports*. 2003 Jul–Aug; **118**(4): 293–302.

The Cross Cultural Health Care Program video *Communicating Effectively through an Interpreter*. 1998. Available from www.xculture.org

Fernandez A, Schillinger D, Grumbach K, *et al*. Physician language ability and cultural competence: an exploratory study of communication with Spanish-speaking patients. *J Gen Intern Med*. 2004 Feb; **19**(2): 167–74.

Grantmakers In Health. In the right words: addressing language and culture in providing health care. *Issue Brief (Grantmakers Health)*. 2003 Aug; **18**: 1–44.

Ngo-Metzger Q, Massagli MP, Clarridge BR, *et al*. Linguistic and cultural barriers to care. *J Gen Intern Med*. 2003 Jan; **18**(1): 44–52.

Office of Minority Health, US Department of Health and Human Services. National standards for culturally and linguistically appropriate services (CLAS) in health care. *Federal Register*. 2000; **65**(247): 80865–79. Available from: http://www.omhrc.gov/clas/finalcultural1a.htm

SESSION 22 National Standards for Culturally and Linguistically Appropriate Services (CLAS) in Health Care – Language Access Services (Standards 4–7)

4. Health care organizations must offer and provide language assistance services, including bilingual staff and interpreter services, at no cost to each patient/consumer with limited English proficiency, at all points of contact, in a timely manner, during all hours of operation.
5. Health care organizations must provide to patients/consumers in their preferred language both verbal offers and written notices informing them of their right to receive language assistance services.
6. Health care organizations must assure the competence of language assistance provided to limited English proficient patients/consumers by interpreters and bilingual staff. Family and friends should not be used to provide interpretation services (except on request by the patient/consumer).
7. Health care organizations must make available easily understood patient-related materials and post signage in the languages of the commonly encountered groups and/or groups represented in the service area.

SESSION 23 Cultural Knowledge: Discussion of a Selected Cultural Group

Session Description

This is the third annual cultural knowledge session. The intent is for the local program to select one area of interest each year, preferably a cultural group that, while present in the greater community, is not part of the clinical practice of the learners. At the US census website, Quickfact sheets can be obtained for any state or county and many major cities. In addition to groups selected by country or ethnicity, religious groups can also be the focus for a session, again selected to enlarge the knowledge base of the learners. For this session, it is suggested that a small group of learners (e.g., a class of residents) be assigned to develop and deliver this session.

Session Objectives

After participation in the session, learners should be better able to:
1. value the importance of diversity in health care and address the challenges and opportunities it poses (Objective 3 – attitude)
2. describe historical models of common health beliefs (for example, illness in the context of 'hot and cold'), and identify questions about health practices and beliefs that might be important in a specific local community (Objective 7 – knowledge)
3. discuss race, ethnicity, and culture in the context of the medical interview and health care. Exhibit comfort when conversing with patients/colleagues about cultural issues (Objective 9 – attitude, skill)
4. describe methods to identify key community leaders. Describe strategies for partnering with community activists to eliminate racism and other bias from health care. Collaborate to address community needs (Objective 28 – knowledge, skill).

Instructional Materials

Presentation outline, distributed some weeks prior to the presentation date; materials requested by learners to facilitate presentations (a list of potential resources is given in Sessions 3 and 13); session objectives; small group activity; commitment to change forms or index cards.

Time Schedule

00:00 – 00:05   Session introduction
00:05 – 00:20   Presentation of stimulus materials (interview with community member or leader, video clip, panel, quiz/trivia contest, case presentation, etc. – *see* openers in Section 4)
00:20 – 00:40   Formal presentation of information (*see* outline)
00:40 – 00:55   Small group activities: group discussion in relation to a) implications for care of patients; b) community resources; and c) how learners might collaborate with community leaders to address needs
00:55 – 01:00   Session summary and portfolio entry (commitment to change)

Process

Distribute presentation assignment and guidelines (*see* below) some weeks prior to the presentation date. Instructors will want to work with the groups of learners in preparing their presentation, particularly if this is their first experience.
1. Session introduction (5 minutes): the instructor can introduce the topic and its place in the overall curriculum and then turn the session over to the students/residents in charge or move directly to the introductory activity.
2. Introductory activity (15 minutes): as selected by the learners presenting.
3. Formal presentation of information (15–20 minutes): the formal presentation of information can be done using PowerPoint or provided in a handout. PowerPoint allows insertion of a short video clip, photos, quiz items, etc. for the audience. *See* the attached outline for a overview of the materials to cover if the focus is a cultural group (e.g. African-Americans,

Hispanics), people from a specific country (e.g. Mexico, China), or a specific religious heritage (e.g. Muslim, Buddhist).

4. Small group activity (15–20 minutes): a minimum of 15 minutes should be scheduled for this activity selected by the presenting learners.

5. Conclusion and portfolio entry (5 minutes): the instructor should thank the learners and request that they place a copy of their work in their portfolios. All learners (presenters and audience) should complete a commitment to change form and place them in their portfolios. Encourage learners to apply new knowledge and insights directly in their clinical work.

Cautionary Note

It is important to emphasize that knowledge learning about other groups helps health care providers develop hypotheses about the cultural background of patients. In the end, providers must strive to hold stereotyping 'at bay' and draw conclusions based on information provided by the patient himself/herself.

SESSION 23 HANDOUT Cultural Knowledge Presentation Preparation Guidelines

Directions: the portion of the session you will lead will be 50 minutes in length. If you are working in groups of four or more you may want to divide the tasks and work in pairs. A sample demographic sheet and a resource list are provided for you to use in finding appropriate data and resources. Think of dividing your session into three parts – introductory activity, formal presentation, and small group activity/discussion. Review the description of the session and be sure you understand the session objectives and time schedule.

1. Plan an **introductory activity** (5–15 minutes): the activity should draw the learners toward the topic and make them ready (if not eager) to learn more about the cultural group. Be creative – make it fun for your learners as well as educational. Potential methods include: interview with community member or leader, video clip/debriefing, panel, quiz/trivia contest (using teams, audience response system, or paper and pencil), case presentation, etc. In the Video Resources section (Section 7) there are several sources that provide relevant clips including brief segments from the *Worlds Apart* tapes (Laotian child, African-American man, Mexican-American woman, and Muslim man). **Caution**: if a video is used it should focus the audience on the objectives for this session.

2. Plan and rehearse the **formal presentation** (20 minutes). You may want a handout to accompany your PowerPoint presentation to expand on important areas. The PowerPoint presentation should focus on the things most relevant to health beliefs, health disparities, and health care disparities. The talk might be divided into three parts that can be divided equally or with more time spent on the last two sections.

    Overview (6 minutes)
    a) *Country* – language, including number of dialects; any important interpersonal relationships (e.g. naming, status, roles, greetings, displays of respect, general etiquette); unique information about marriage, family kinship (marriage, gender roles, extended families); religious beliefs and practices.
    b) *Ethnic Group* – same information as for country with addition of countries of origin.
    c) *Religious Group* – basic tenants in relevant areas of daily living.

    Health beliefs and practices (7 minutes)
    Described in general or in relation to relevant topics like: a) reproduction (pregnancy, child birth, post partum practices); b) nutrition and food; c) alcohol, drugs, tobacco; d) attitudes toward death and suffering; and e) complementary therapies.

    Disparities and community resources (7 minutes)
    Discuss any data on health disparities in your community, state, or in the nation and provide information about local community leader(s) and community groups/resources serving this community.

3. **Small group activity** (15 minutes): a minimum of 15 minutes should be scheduled for this activity. Divide the learners into small groups to apply the information provided in the presentation. If the whole group is relatively small, use three groups; assign one item to each group (5–7 minutes). Sample items are: a) implications of the culturally based health beliefs of this group for care of patients; b) community resources for this cultural group; and c) how learners might collaborate with community leaders to address needs. Suggest that the groups agree on three to five items to share. In the follow-up discussion with the entire group, the facilitator should address all three items. Seek input from each group (8–10 minutes).

SESSION 24 Health Care Policy and the Role of the Clinician

Session Description

The elimination of health disparities may ultimately depend on social policy (e.g. the CLAS Standards). Health care providers can play an important role in the development and implementation of health policy that addresses justice in the health care arena. This session provides an overview of health policy at all levels and allows for participants to explore ways they may serve as powerful advocates in the health policy arena. This session will be enhanced by inviting a local expert in health policy and clinician empowerment to serve as a guest lecturer. Commitment to change can serve as a thoughtful and helpful conclusion to the presentation.

Session Objectives

After participation in the session, learners should be better able to:

1. value the importance of social determinants (e.g. education, culture, socioeconomic status, housing, and employment) and community factors on health and strive to address them (Objective 6 – attitude, skills)
2. describe the role of government and health policy in the arena of health disparities and culturally responsive medicine (Objective 19 – knowledge)
3. describe methods to identify key community leaders; describe strategies for partnering with community activists to eliminate racism and other bias from health care through policy development. Collaborate to address community needs (Objective 28 – knowledge, skills)
4. discuss potential roles clinicians may take to advocate for patients on both an individual level as well as on a larger policy level and play a role in advocacy for justice in patient care (systems based practice, skills).

Instructional Materials

Identify and invite a local guest speaker on this topic, if available. If no speaker is available, you may want to bring a story of how policies have helped and/or hindered work to diminish health and health care disparities (access, quality, cost); commitment to change forms.

Time Schedule

00:00 – 00:05   Session introduction
00:05 – 00:35   Guest presentation on health policy and the role of the clinician
00:35 – 00:50   Small group activity
00:50 – 01:00   Commitment to change and session conclusion

Process

1. Session introduction (5 minutes): the session introduction serves as an opportunity to introduce presenter and participants. Moreover, it is the opportunity to present the session objectives to the learners, and explain how this session is part of the larger culturally responsive care curriculum.
2. Formal presentation – guest speaker (30 minutes): guest presenter should provide a historical overview of health policy in the arena of health disparities elimination, as well as current and future trends. It can be helpful to provide descriptions of clinicians who have been key advocates in policy development as role models for the participants. Encourage the speaker to actively engage the learners with challenges, cases, and/or questions via an audience response system.
3. Small group activity (15 minutes): select a current issue and present the learners with a challenge to consider it in relation to policies or laws that have been suggested by policy makers (e.g. universal health care). Guide the learners through identifying key stakeholders and underlying ethical principles, as well as thinking about risks and benefits of the options.
4. Commitment to change and session conclusion (10 minutes): participants are asked to

note at least one thing they will do to increase their participation in the larger community (advocacy, policy work, etc.). Conclude with a review of the session's goals and central learning points.

Cautionary Notes

Finding the best expert presenter in this area may take some preparation time. It will be important to work closely with the presenter regarding the time frame (30 minutes, including time for questions and answers/discussion) and the content of the talk, so that it meets the objectives for the session.

Resources

Baquet CR, Carter-Pokras O, Bengen-Seltzer B. Healthcare disparities and models for change. *Am J Manag Care*. 2004; **10**(Special Issue): SP5–11.

Bloche MG. Health care disparities: science, politics, and race. *N Eng J Med*. 2004 Apr 8; **350**(15): 1568–70.

Exworthy M, Washington AE. Organizational strategies to tackle health-care disparities in the USA. *Health Serv Manag Res*. 2006 Feb; **19**(1): 44–51.

Unnatural Causes (website includes activities and resources): www.unnaturalcauses.org

SESSION 25 Disparities Related to Gender

Session Description

This session allows learners to increase their knowledge of the extent of gender disparities in health and health care, as well as deepen their understanding of the reasons behind these disparities. The session concludes with a commitments exercise aimed at empowering the learners to take an active role in eliminating gender disparities.

Session Objectives

After participation in this session, learners should be better able to:
1. recognize and describe how access, historical, political, environmental and institutional factors (including racism and discrimination) impact health and underlie health and health care disparities (Objective 17 – attitudes, knowledge)
2. identify and discuss key areas of disparities described in *Healthy People 2010* and the IOM Report, *Unequal Treatment* that relate to gender; discuss barriers to eliminating these health disparities (Objective 18 – knowledge)
3. identify and discuss the contributors to disparities (patient, provider, health care system and society) and discuss the challenges and barriers to eliminating health disparities (Objective 19 – knowledge)
4. describe patterns of health care disparities that can result, at least in part, from clinician bias, recognize disparities that are amenable to intervention and value eliminating disparities (Objective 20 – attitudes, knowledge).

Instructional Materials

The poem *Maria* by Rafael Campo; data sheets printed from the National Women's Law Center 2004 Report Card.

Time Schedule

00:00 – 00:15 Session introduction: *Maria* poem and narrative writing
00:15 – 00:30 Data review: *Making the Grade on Women's Health: A National and State-by-State Report Card*
00:30 – 00:40 Think-write-share
00:40 – 00:55 Group brainstorm: reasons for gender disparities
00:50 – 00:55 Session conclusion, portfolio with commitment to change

Process

1. Session introduction (15 minutes): the session will open with a reading of the poem *Maria* by Rafael Campo. Read the poem aloud twice to the group and ask them to complete a brief narrative writing assignment. Ask the learners to take five minutes to write from the point of view of the patient. The writing should go into the learner's portfolio. Allow one person to share their narrative. Then, move the discussion to the topic of gender-based health disparities.
2. Data review (15 minutes): allow participants to review data from the National Women's Law Center: *Making the Grade on Women's Health: A National and State-by-State Report Card* (see Section 7 for more details). The report from your state plus the fact sheet on 'Low-Income Women's Access to Care' and/or 'Racial and Ethnic Disparities in Health Care' should be sufficient. Have a set of questions prepared to help guide their review. Suggest that they write down their answers. Example questions:
   a) State report: how do you interpret our state's grade and rank? In comparison to other states, in which area do we excel? In which area are we far behind?
   b) Low-income women's access: what are the primary barriers to access nationally? In our local community?
   c) Racial and ethnic disparities: what are the primary issues nationally? In our state?
3. Think-write-share (10 minutes): the learners have completed the 'think' and 'write' portions, now allow participants to share their reflections and observations about the data they have studied with a partner or small group and then briefly with the entire group.

4. Discussion and brainstorm (15 minutes): having looked at the data, and reviewed the poem/case example, it is important to engage the group in a thoughtful discussion of reasons for the observed gender disparities. These can be elicited according to the categories described in Session 4: the patient, the providers, the health care system, and society.
5. Session conclusion, portfolio with commitment to change (5 minutes): each learner should complete their commitment to reflect on one thing they can do to help eliminate gender-based health disparities as health providers specifically, and as citizens more generally.

Cautionary Note

When discussing the data on gender health disparities, it is worth raising the question, to what degree the data reflect gender disparities *per se*, or are reflective of generally poor health conditions and care for the US population as a whole.

Resources

Campo R. *What the Body Told*. Durham, NC: Duke University Press; 1996. p. 70.

Clark A, Fong C, Jacobs MR. Health disparities among US women of color: an overview. Presented at the Institute of Women's Health Margaret E. Mahoney Annual Symposium *Health Disparities Among Women of Color*; 2002 Apr 16; Washington, DC. Available from: www.jiwh.org

Gregory K, Peck MG, Davidson EC. Pregnancy and women's health. In: Satcher D, Pamies R, editors. *Multicultural Medicine and Health Disparities*. New York: McGraw-Hill; 2006. pp. 105–26

Institute of Medicine. *Women and Health Research: ethical and legal issues of including women in clinical studies*, vol. 1; 1994. Available from: www.nap.edu/catalog.php?record_ID=2304

National Women's Law Center. *Making the Grade on Women's Health: A national and state-by-state report card*; 2004. Available from: http://www.nwlc.org/details.cfm?id=1861&section=health

SESSION 26 Building Cultural Skills: Negotiated Care

Session Description

This session provides learners with the skills to more effectively negotiate treatment plans with patients that incorporate the patient's world view and healing preferences as well as the provider's knowledge and expertise. A standardized patient (SP) exercise will provide practice on negotiating care in the clinical encounter.

Session Objectives

After participation in the session, learners should be better able to:

1. describe models of effective cross-cultural communication, and physician–patient negotiation (Objective 22 – knowledge)
2. demonstrate respect for patients' cultural and health beliefs and use negotiating and problem-solving skills in shared decision-making with a patient. (Objective 23 – attitude, skill)
3. assess and enhance patient adherence based on the patient's explanatory model. Describe ways to enhance patient adherence by collaborating with traditional/community healers (Objective 25 – knowledge, skill).

Instructional Materials

Flip chart and pens; SP and an SP case; student portfolio materials.

Time Schedule

00:00 – 00:05 Session introduction
00:05 – 00:20 Didactic presentation on negotiating skills
00:20 – 00:45 Negotiation with SP
00:45 – 00:50 Brainstorming
00:50 – 01:00 Reflective writing for the portfolio

Process

1. Introduction with best-worst warm-up (5 minutes): the purpose is to focus the learners so this moves very quickly.
   a) One half of the learners: 'Imagine a doctor–patient encounter which is marked by effective negotiation and a mutually agreed upon treatment plan. Take two minutes to make a list of adjectives that describe this scenario.'
   b) The other half of the learners: 'Imagine a doctor–patient encounter in which there is very little agreement between the parties as to the plan for action. Take two minutes to make a list of adjectives that describe this scenario.'
   c) Ask one learner to begin reading the positive list aloud, go around quickly until there is nothing new to add. Repeat the process for the negative list. Often the learners will note that the negative list reflects an absence of the positive characteristics.
2. Didactic presentation on negotiating skills (15 minutes):
   a) Begin with a quick review of the LEARN mnemonic, which includes negotiation as an important final phase:
      Listen with sympathy and understanding to the patient's perceptions
      Explain your perception of the problem
      Acknowledge and discuss the differences and similarities
      Recommend treatment
      Negotiate agreement
   b) This presentation is based on the book *Getting to Yes: Negotiating Agreement Without Giving In* by Roger Fisher and William Ury. The instructor should read this book in preparation for this presentation and build his/her own medical encounter examples. Fisher and Ury present a four-stage process for coming to a good agreement between parties that is wise, efficient and that improves the parties' relationships. They suggest that traditional bargaining (such as haggling over the use of an advertised drug versus

a generic drug) is inefficient and tends to grow resentments. Principled negotiation, the model they present, has four components or principles.

    i. Separate the people from the issues. This helps each party remove the personal aspect of the dilemma, and to approach a clearer and more substantive view of the problem at hand. For example, instead of a physician and patient arguing about how much to exercise, it may be helpful for both of them to look at the larger issue of inactivity and health.

    ii. Focus on each party's interests rather than their positions. The authors write, 'Your position is something you have decided upon. Your interests are what caused you to so decide' (p. 42). Seek shared basic interests such as security, safety and well-being.

    iii. When the interests have been identified, these can be discussed together, with each explaining him/herself clearly while remaining open to different proposals and positions.

    iv. Generate options. Move away from a win-lose mentality by identifying obstacles to agreement and seeking creative solutions. A quick brainstorm can often dislodge frustration and hopelessness. The authors suggest that, 'optimal solutions are those that are of low cost to you and of high benefit to the other – and vice versa' (p. 79). For the patient who insists on herbal treatments to the exclusion of the physician's prescriptions, the physician may be able to suggest additional herbal preparations (that are safe) along with a trial of the prescription, or as a buffer against potential side effects. Use objective criteria to resolve differences, as opposed to a battle of wills.

    A demonstration with an SP will be a very helpful tool to illustrate this process. Write the four steps on a flip chart page and tape it where all learners can see it.

3. Progressive interview with an SP (25 minutes): the progressive interview uses a time-in/ time-out technique to control the instruction as the learners take turns as the interviewer.

    a) Rules need to be established in terms of who can call a 'time-out'. Generally, only the current 'interviewer' or the instructor can call a time-out (by making a 'T' with his/her two hands). During a time-out the SP bows his/her head and is 'not in the room'. When time-in is called then the patient returns to the point in the interview where the time-out was called with no apparent interruption in the interview.

    b) Once the interview begins, the current interviewer can call time out to ask for advice from the other students. The instructor can call time out to make a point or to change interviewer.

    c) The interview generally moves fairly quickly, no more than a couple of minutes per learner.

    d) After each learner (or about five learners if the group is large) has had an opportunity to interview the SP, the instructor leads a discussion of the process and the main learning points. Learners may provide feedback to each other as time permits.

4. Quick brainstorm (5 minutes): ask the group to identify and call out additional areas (outside of the doctor-patient encounter) in the practice of medicine and in their personal lives where negotiating skills would be useful.

5. Reflective writing for the portfolio (10 minutes): think about one specific patient encounter where you were frustrated with your inability to negotiate an optimal patient care plan. Re-write history using the negotiation steps presented today. Write a new, positive dialogue with the patient. Place the writing in your portfolio.

Resources

Botelho R. A negotiation model for the doctor-patient relationship. *Fam Pract.* 1992; **9**(2): 210–18.

Bregman B, Irvine C. Subjectifying the patient: creative writing and the clinical encounter. *Fam Med.* 2004; **36**(6): 400–1.

Charon R. Narrative medicine: a model for empathy, reflection, profession and trust. *JAMA.* 2001; **286**: 1897–902.

Fisher R, Ury W. *Getting to Yes: Negotiation agreement without giving in.* New York: Penguin Books; 1983.

Levin SJ, Like RC, Gottlieb JC. Useful clinical interviewing mnemonics. *Patient Care.* 2000; **34**: 189–90.

Quality Care for Diverse Populations, video with Instruction booklet. Kansas City, MO: American Academy of Family Physicians; 2002.

Potential Beginning for an SP Negotiation (Case 1)

The physician receives this information: patient is 79 years old and doesn't exercise, despite obesity, diabetes and hypertension.

The patient receives this information: you are 79 years old and don't exercise, despite obesity, diabetes and hypertension. You have not 'walked daily in the neighborhood' as prescribed by the physician at the last session because your neighborhood is not safe, you are responsible for providing childcare for grandchildren, and it has been very cold lately.

Potential Beginning for an SP Negotiation (Case 2)

The physician receives this information: patient is a 40-year-old parent demanding antibiotics for their sick child. You do not feel these medications are warranted.

The patient receives this information: you are a 40-year-old parent demanding antibiotics for their sick child. You remember that your own mother died from a terrible infection that went untreated by her physician.

SESSION 27 Teaching Cultural Competence to Others: Twenty-Eight Objectives, Five Types of Teaching Techniques

Session Overview

In this session we familiarize the learners with a number of techniques that they have experienced in the Cultural Competence Curriculum. Several instructional techniques are deconstructed, providing learners with a deepened understanding of the use of these instructional strategies to bolster their own capacity to teach cultural medicine in the future.

Session Objectives

After participation in the session, learners should be better able to:
1. value the importance of curiosity, empathy, and respect in patient care and the importance of continuous growth as a healer (Objective 11 – attitudes)
2. discuss the Cultural Competence Curriculum and its core principles
3. value teaching cultural competence to other physicians and health care professionals, health professions' students, and hospital/clinical staff
4. describe at least three teaching techniques that can be used to add interaction and/or depth to cultural competence curricula.

Instructional Materials

Handouts: curriculum overview and teaching techniques overview; flip chart and markers; optional – bring two copies of this book for the learners to examine.

Time Schedule

00:00 – 00:05   Session introduction
00:05 – 00:20   Review curriculum and objectives
00:20 – 00:55   Teaching techniques
00:55 – 01:00   Portfolio and session conclusion

Process

1. Session introduction (5 minutes): this session uses a challenge as an opener. 'You have joined a practice. Since you are a graduate of a program with a strong cultural competence curriculum, you have been charged with developing training for the other providers. Take one minute and list as many things as you can think of that you would want to include in such a program. Base it on your experience of the provider needs, and on what you have learned thus far in this curriculum.' Use brainstorming to gather the input quickly on to a flip chart or projection system. If the group is small (less than 20), use the formal process of going around the room, allowing each person to add one until there are no more to add. Before you begin, remind the group of the rules of brainstorming – no judgment, all ideas are acceptable at this point.
2. Review of curriculum (15 minutes): distribute the two-page overview of the curriculum, attached to this session. Provide a few minutes to read it. Use facilitation to guide them to seeing the similarities and differences between their list and the objectives of this curriculum.
3. Teaching techniques (35 minutes): provide the one-page handout on teaching techniques.
   a) Discuss the five types of techniques used in this curriculum. You might remind learners that all positive (or negative) behaviors require four things: sufficient knowledge (know how), adequate skill (able to do), awareness/attitude (recognition that the action should be done and willingness to do it), and environment (that encourages positive behaviors or allows negative behaviors). This curriculum is not just about knowledge – it promotes permanent positive change in practice behaviors, meaning that techniques cannot be superficial (skill builders only). To reach higher we have to ask more (catalysts and intensifiers) of learners and even make them uncomfortable at times (5 minutes).

b) If this resonates with them, let them discuss how some techniques make them uncomfortable. Just remember that the curriculum uses a wide variety of techniques, in recognition of differing readiness, personalities and learning styles (5 minutes).

c) Ask them to identify any techniques they recognize from the curriculum to date, or any special skills (or lack thereof) that they have noted from the course directors or instructors. For those identified techniques, ask the group if they have any questions about the technique and be ready to discuss. Be sure you are very familiar with the teaching techniques used to date in Year 3 (5 minutes).

d) Briefly discuss the three techniques used so far in this session – openers, brainstorming and facilitation (5 minutes).

e) Activity: take the opportunity to demonstrate two more techniques (15 minutes).

   i. Narrative writing: 'Take the next five minutes and write two paragraphs. In the first write about your favorite learning technique from the list of 21. Describe why you prefer it above all others. In the second paragraph describe your least favorite technique. What about it makes you uncomfortable, angry or dissatisfied with it?'

   ii. Think-pair-share: 'After you are done you will share your reflections with a partner. As a pair you may then choose to share with the entire group.' After five minutes, have the pairs do the sharing. Do not debrief with the group, but instead discuss the two techniques.

4. Portfolio and session conclusion (5 minutes): briefly review the session objectives and take any questions. Have them complete their commitment to change and place it in their portfolio.

Notes to Instructor

If there are different teaching techniques you would like to highlight, you can substitute relevant activities in 3e in place of the ones suggested. The explanations for each technique are found in Section 4. Resources for teaching techniques, sessions, and exercises are included within each section with many listed in Section 7.

SESSION 27 – HANDOUT 1 Curriculum Overview

Design

This curriculum has been designed as a three-year, 33-hour longitudinal curriculum in cultural competence and culturally responsive medicine. The learning objectives and training modules are linked to the Core Competencies delineated by the Accreditation Council for Graduate Medical Education (ACGME – available from www.acgme.org) and the Association of American Medical Colleges (AAMC) as reflected in the Tool for Assessing Cultural Competence Training (TAACT – available from http://www.aamc.org/meded/tacct/ culturalcomped.pdf). At the conclusion of training, learners will have received ample training and experience in the awareness/attitudes, knowledge and skills components of culturally responsive care.

Delivery

The curriculum is like an ever-spinning carousel. New residents get on each year, but as long as they stay three years, they will receive the entire training. The curriculum begins with three introductory sessions (Sessions A, B, and C), which are presented as part of intern orientation. These sessions provide learners with the basics necessary to 'join' the three-year curriculum already in progress for the second and third year residents. There are three parallel but not repeating annual cycles. For example, the content for Session 1 each year is novel yet reinforces the learning of previous Session 1 material.

The annual 10-session program follows the following agenda:

Sessions A, B, C	Introduction to basic concepts
Session 1	Bias, power and the doctor–patient relationship
Session 2	Developing culturally competent communication skills
Session 3	Cultural knowledge of selected cultural groups (country, ethnicity, religion)
Session 4	Socio-cultural and political aspects
Session 5	Special populations (GLBTQ, elderly, women)
Session 6	Effective communication: negotiation skills
Session 7	Cultural issues in teaching and research
Session 8	Annual review of health disparity data – selected topics
Session 9	Resident presentations of own cases
Session 10	Annual review of progress

Curricular material can be adapted for different teaching needs and schedules (e.g. a semester course).

Following is a table of objectives by Unit in the curriculum, and the sessions in which each is addressed.

No.	Objectives	Sessions
	Unit I. Introduction to Culture and Cultural Competence	
1	Define, in contemporary terms, race, ethnicity, and culture, and their implications in health care.	A, 1,11
2	Become aware of their own cultural heritage, gender, class, ethnic-racial identity, sexual orientation, disability, age, and spirituality; be able to reflect on it and describe it.	B, 10, 20, 30
3	Value the importance of diversity in health care and address the challenges/opportunities it poses.	A, C, 3, 13, 14, 23
4	Identify patterns of national data on health, health care disparities, and quality of health care, and be able to discuss.	8, 18, 28
5	Discuss the epidemiology of health and health care disparities for the local community using *Healthy People 2010* and other resources.	8, 18, 28

No.	Objectives	Sessions
	Unit II. Key Concepts in Cultural Competence	
6	Value the importance of social determinants (e.g. education, culture, socioeconomic status, housing, and employment) and community factors on health and strive to address them.	C, 24
7	Describe historical models of common health beliefs and identify questions about health practices and beliefs that might be important in a specific local community.	3, 9, 13, 19, 23, 29
8	Identify healing traditions and beliefs of patients and/or their families, including ethno-medical beliefs. Elicit patient preferences, listen and respond appropriately to patient feedback about key cross-cultural issues. Elicit additional information about ethno-medical conditions and ethno-medical healers.	B, 6, 9, 12, 19, 29
9	Discuss race, ethnicity, and culture in the context of the medical interview and health care. Exhibit comfort when conversing with patients/colleagues about cultural issues.	B, 3, 7, 12, 13, 17, 23
10	Recognize and describe institutional cultural issues for own institution.	14, 22
11	Value the importance of curiosity, empathy, and respect in patient care and the importance of continuous growth as a healer.	7, 17
	Unit III. Bias, Stereotyping, Culture and Clinical Decision-making	
12	Recognize their own potential for bias and stereotyping, be able to identify their own stereotypes and biases and explore how their attitudes, biases and stereotypes affect clinical encounters, clinical decision-making and quality of care.	1, 10, 11, 20, 21, 30
13	Identify and appreciate how clinician bias and stereotyping can affect interactions with patients, families, communities, and other members of the health care team, and the link between effective communication and quality care.	1, 11
14	Describe the impact of the patient's context (cultural heritage, gender, class, ethnic-racial identity, sexual orientation, disability, age, and spirituality) on clinical decision-making.	7, 17
15	Describe strategies for reducing own biases, and those of others; demonstrate strategies to assess, manage, and reduce bias and its effects in clinical encounters and in clinical practice.	10, 20, 21, 30
16	Describe the inherent power imbalance between physician and patient and how it affects the clinical encounter.	21
	Unit IV. Health and Health Care Disparities	
17	Recognize and describe how access, historical, political, environmental, and institutional factors (including racism and discrimination) impact health and underlie health and health care disparities.	4, 5, 15, 25
18	Identify how race, ethnicity, and social determinants of health (e.g. education, culture, housing, socioeconomic status, and employment) affect health and health care quality, cost, and outcomes.	4, 5, 15, 25
19	Identify and discuss the contributors to disparities (patient, provider, health care system, and society) and discuss the challenges and barriers to eliminating health disparities.	4, 24, 25
20	Describe patterns of health care disparities that can result, at least in part, from clinician bias, recognize disparities that are amenable to intervention and value eliminating disparities.	4, 5, 10, 15, 20, 25, 30
21	Describe systemic and medical-encounter issues related to health care disparities, including communication issues, clinical decision-making, and patient preferences.	5, 11, 14, 15
	Unit V. Cultural Competence in Patient Care	
22	Describe models of effective cross-cultural communication, assessment, and physician–patient negotiation and identify common challenges in cross-cultural communication (e.g. trust, style).	2, 9, 16, 19, 26, 29
23	Conduct and document a culturally responsive history and physical examination within the context of family-centered care. Elicit a cultural, social, and medical history, including a patient's health beliefs/model of their illness. Use negotiating and problem-solving skills in shared decision-making.	2, 12, 16, 22, 26
24	Describe the functions of an interpreter and effective ways of working with an interpreter. Identify when an interpreter is needed and collaborate effectively with an interpreter.	22
25	Assess and enhance patient adherence based on the patient's explanatory model. Describe ways to enhance patient adherence by collaborating with traditional/community healers.	9, 19, 26, 29
26	Critically appraise the literature as it relates to health disparities, including systems issues and quality in health care.	8, 18, 28

cont.

No.	Objectives	Sessions
	Unit VI. Cultural Competence and Community Action	
27	Describe factors that contribute to variability in population health; outline a framework to assess communities according to population health criteria, social mores, cultural beliefs, and needs.	C
28	Describe methods to identify key community leaders; describe strategies for partnering to eliminate racism and other bias from health care; collaborate to address community needs.	3, 13, 23, 24

SESSION 27 – HANDOUT 2 Teaching Techniques – Overview

The teaching techniques described and used in the Cultural Competence Curriculum have been organized into the following five categories.

Attention Grabbers: these techniques open up a topic, grab the learners' attention and help them to focus on the issue under study.
1. Brainstorming and best-worst warm-up
2. Openers and closers
3. Video clips

Skill Builders: these techniques are used to help learners gain an initial awareness and knowledge in relation to a topic, and/or to build the core communication and interaction skills needed to provide culturally responsive care.
4. Expanded cases and conferences – expanded to emphasize cultural issues
5. Formal presentation (lecture and demonstration)
6. Independent study using written or technology-based materials
7. Role play
8. Standardized patients
9. Teaching objective structured clinical examination (OSCE)

Catalysts: these techniques are used to stimulate active learning in small or large groups and help ensure that learners are interacting with the concepts presented and with each other.
10. Progressive disclosure cases – cases presented with stopping points for discussion
11. Quizzes, games, polls, audience response system
12. Small group activities – discussion and task-based activities to encourage active learning
13. Think-write-share – actively engages learners in interaction with challenging issues

Intensifiers: the skilled instructor uses these techniques to encourage learners to greater depth of awareness and knowledge and intends to encourage positive change within the learner, and in their practice performance.
14. Commitment to change – learners commit to changes that take learning into practice
15. Debriefing – skilled guidance following an activity to extract maximum learning from it
16. Facilitation – skills in guiding interactive discussion, particularly on controversial topics
17. Narrative and reflective writing
18. Student/resident presentations

Trackers: these tools are used to track learners across time and encourage continuing growth.
19. Journal – ongoing collection of writings
20. Portfolio – collection of a variety of selected learner-generated products
21. Reflection and self-assessment – periodic review of one's own progress toward goals

SESSION 28 Focused Review of Local, State, and National Health Data (Diseases)

Session Description

This annual session (sessions 8, 18, and 28) is designed to provide the opportunity for learners to review actual health status data: national, state and particularly local. In the state of California, data is provided annually that compares each county with all other counties, with the state average, and with the *Healthy People 2010* goal for a variety of health issues. This data should be reviewed (check you own state Department of Health for similar data) along with any data collected in relation to PBLI (practice-based learning and improvement) goals for your program's clinic or hospital. Learners may also be able to look at the data on their own patient population in relation to program goals or *Healthy People 2010* goals. *Healthy People 2010* is a very extensive document addressing a wide variety of issues. Familiarity with both it and the *Healthy People Midcourse Review* will increase understanding of the goals and the progress from 2000 to 2005.

Session Objectives

After participation in the session, learners should be better able to:
1. identify patterns of national data on health, health care disparities, and quality of health care, and describe them in a worldwide immigration context (Objective 4 – knowledge)
2. discuss the epidemiology of health and health care disparities for the local community using *Healthy People 2010* and other resources (Objective 5 – knowledge, skill)
3. critically appraise the literature as it relates to health disparities, including systems issues and quality in health care (Objective 26 – skill).

Instructional Materials

National, regional and *Healthy People 2010* data (copies made for each person or each small group); local hospital, clinic and individual resident data if available; small group assignments for this session based on the data focus selected.

Time Schedule

00:00 – 00:05   Session introduction
00:05 – 00:30   Small group data review
00:30 – 00:50   Facilitation of group discussion of common themes
00:50 – 01:00   Conclusion of session, portfolio with commitment to change

Process
Prior to Session
    a) Select the topic for data review from those included in *Healthy People 2010*. Select a topic that resonates with the local community. Below are several suggestions – our suggestion for Session 28 is diabetes.
    b) Plan a relevant small group assignment that requires the students/residents to review the data in a meaningful manner (generally a series of questions to answer, see sample assignment).
1. Introduction (5 minutes): this session should begin with an opener that draws the learners' attention to the focus of the session. A quote or a statistic could open the session, or the learners could be presented with a challenge in relation to health care within the clinic, health center or community where data would be important in addressing an issue.
2. Small group exercises – data review (25 minutes): provide the pre-planned assignment to each group along with the data sheets prepared in advance. Monitor the progress of the groups and provide assistance in examining the data if required.
3. Debriefing of exercise and discussion of challenges and common themes (20 minutes): use facilitation to debrief the exercise. Be careful to include all groups in reporting the answers to the questions in your pre-planned exercise. For each question, ask a different group to provide their answer first. Ask all groups for any other additional or differing

interpretations and ideas. Encourage the students to discuss any disagreements. Return to the data if necessary.
4. Session conclusion and journal (10 minutes): learners should be asked how they might make use of data in their own practices. Ask them to commit to making just one change over this next year in relation to use of data to enhance their evidence-based practice.

Data Sources

Agency for Health Care Quality and Research: http://www.ahrq.gov/qual/measurix.htm
On this website, you will find two reports: 1. the annual National Healthcare Disparities Reports (NHDR) examining the distribution of improvement in health care quality; and 2. the National Healthcare Quality Report (NHQR), addressing the current state of health care quality.

California Center for Health Statistics: http://www.dhs.ca.gov/hisp/chs/OHIR/reports/
This site provides a wide variety of data reports related to the health status of Californians. Of particular interest are the annual County Health Status Profiles that provide comparative data for all California counties in relation to each other and to the *Healthy People 2010* goals. Other data include deaths by zip code, and statistics for many disease states and causes of death.

Centers for Disease Control Office of Minority Health: http://www.cdc.gov/omh/AboutUs/disparities.htm
Obtain data on health disparities at the Center for Disease Control.

DHHS Office of Minority Health Resource Center: http://www.omhrc.gov/
This site has information in three categories: staying healthy, health disparities, and communities in action.

Healthy People 2010: http://www.healthypeople.gov/Document/tableofcontents.htm
Healthy People 2010 provides a large set of health objectives for the nation to achieve by the year 2010. The *Healthy People Midcourse Review* reports progress toward meeting the *Healthy People 2010* goals: http://www.healthypeople.gov/data/midcourse/default.htm#pubs

Kaiser Family Foundation – State Health Facts: http://www.statehealthfacts.org/cgi-bin/healthfacts.cgi
This site provides free, up-to-date, and easy-to-use health data on over 500 health topics for all 50 states.

National Center for Health Statistics: www.cdc.gov/nchs/data/hus/hus06.pdf
Health, United States 2006, with Chartbook on Trends in the Health of Americans provides data for the United States in comparison to other nations and a wide variety of health data and comparisons including those by race, ethnicity, gender, and age. Downloads as a PDF document.

SESSION 28 Focused Review of Local, State, and National Health Data

Sample Data Sources for Diseases

1. 2007 County Health Status Profiles for the state of California: http://www.dhs.ca.gov/hisp/chs/OHIR/reports/

All cancer deaths	pages 5–6
Colorectal (colon) cancer	pages 7–8
Lung cancer	pages 9–10
Female breast cancer	pages 11–12
Diabetes	pages 15–16
Coronary heart disease	pages 19–20
Cerebrovascular disease (stroke)	pages 21–22

2. National Center for Health Statistics. *Health, United States, 2007 With Chartbook on Trends in the Health of Americans.* http://www.cdc.gov/nchs/data/hus/hus07.pdf
   - Death rates by race/ethnicity: diseases of the heart (Table 36); cerebrovascular diseases (Table 37); all malignant neoplasms (Table 38); neoplasms of the breast (Table 40).
   - Determinants and measures of health: cancer incidence rates (Table 53); five-year cancer survival rates (Table 54); diabetes among adults (Table 55); cigarette smoking (Tables 63–65); hypertension (Table 69); serum total cholesterol levels (Table 70); overweight/obese (Table 73).

3. In California, *Healthy People 2010* objectives. http://www.dhs.ca.gov/chs/OHIR/hp2010/hc2010progress.htm
   Focus Area 3: Cancer; Focus Area 5: Diabetes; Focus Area 12: Heart Disease and Stroke; Focus Area 19: Nutrition and Overweight.

4. *National Healthcare Quality Report*, 2006. http://www.ahrq.gov/qual/measurix.htm
   Effectiveness: Cancer – pages 27–31, Diabetes – pages 32–6, Heart Disease – pages 41–8.

5. *National Healthcare Disparities Report*, 2006. http://www.ahrq.gov/qual/measurix.htm
   Effectiveness: Cancer – pages 36–8, Diabetes – pages 39–42, Heart Disease – pages 45–9.
   Special populations: Racial and ethnic minorities – pages 127–47.

Resources

Albarran NB, Ballesteros MN, Morales GG, *et al*. Dietary behavior and type 2 diabetes care. *Patient Educ Couns*. 2006 May; **61**(2): 191–9.

Brown SA, Blozis SA, Kouzekanani K, *et al*. Dosage effects of diabetes self-management education for Mexican Americans: the Starr County Border Health Initiative. *Diabetes Care*. 2005 Mar; **28**(3): 527–32.

Centers for Disease Control and Prevention (CDC). Racial/ethnic disparities in prevalence, treatment, and control of hypertension – United States, 1999–2002. *MMWR Morb Mortal Wkly Rep*. 2005 Jan 14; **54**(1): 7–9.

Chakraborty BM, Mueller WH, Reeves R, *et al*. For the patient. The importance of health behaviors for better heart health: migration history, health behaviors, and cardiovascular disease risk factors in overweight Mexican-American women. *Ethn Dis*. 2003; **13**(1): 152.

Clark LT. Issues in minority health: atherosclerosis and coronary heart disease in African Americans. *Med Clin North Am*. 2005 Sep; **89**(5): 977–1001, 994.

Holt P. Challenges and strategies: weight management in type 2 diabetes. *Br J Community Nurs*. 2006 Sep; **11**(9): 376–80.

Schulman KA, Berlin JA, Harless W, *et al*. The effect of race and sex on physicians' recommendations for cardiac catheterization. *N Engl J Med*. 1999; **340**: 618–26.

Tan MY. The relationship of health beliefs and complication prevention behaviors of Chinese individuals with type 2 diabetes mellitus. *Diabetes Res Clin Pract*. 2004 Oct; **66**(1): 71–7.

Yancy CW. The prevention of heart failure in minority communities and discrepancies in health care delivery systems. *Med Clin North Am*. 2004 Sep; **88**(5): 1347–68, xii–xiii.

SESSION 28 Focused Review of Local, State, and National Health Data

Diseases/Health Problems

Sample Small Group Assignment

Directions: diabetes is a major health problem. As part of your Practice-Based Learning and Improvement, you will want to track the health of your diabetic patients, as well as their mortality and morbidity. However, in order to understand what your data means you need comparison data from local, region, state and/or national sources.

1. According the 2007 County Health Status Profiles for the State of California, how well is Los Angeles county doing in relation to other counties (and in comparison to Healthy People 2010 goals) in the area of deaths due to diabetes?
2. Look further in the National Center for Health Statistics, *Health, United States, 2007 With Chartbook on Trends in the Health of Americans* for the areas of diabetes among adults (Table 55); and overweight/obese (Table 73). What are the differences, if any, by ethnicity/race among the groups nationally? In California? If available, how does our local data compare?
3. Take a look at some other data sources:
   a) National Healthcare Quality Report, 2007, Section on Diabetes, for California. http://www.ahrq.gov/qual/measurix.htm
   b) National Healthcare Disparities Report, 2007, Section on Diabetes. http://www.ahrq.gov/qual/measurix.htm
   c) Healthy California 2010, Focus Area 5, Diabetes; Focus Area 19: Nutrition and Overweight.

How is the State of California doing in relation to the indicators used regarding Diabetes and Overweight? Where do we excel? What needs more work?

SESSION 29 Annual Second Year Resident Patient Case Presentations: Cultural Issues in Negotiated Care

Session Description
This annual session (sessions 9, 19, and 29) is an application and integration exercise for second year residents to use the materials learned in the cultural competence curriculum up to this point. (With other learners this activity would be non-repeating and occur at the end of Unit V). The expanded case format is used, with relevant cultural issues discussed. Each presenter will have prepared a brief description of a patient case where the patient's health beliefs were an issue in negotiating a care plan. The learner should demonstrate knowledge of the patient, and of any relevant historical model of health beliefs. Learners should be encouraged to include cases where alternative or ethno-medical healers were incorporated. Approximately five to seven learners can share within a one-hour session. Small groups with faculty group leaders can be used to allow more learners to present within a single session.

Session Objectives
After participation in the session, learners should be better able to:
1. describe historical models of common health beliefs (for example, illness in the context of 'hot and cold'), and identify questions about health practices and beliefs that might be important in a specific local community (Objective 7 – knowledge)
2. identify healing traditions and beliefs of patients and/or their families, including ethno-medical beliefs, and describe (Objective 8 – skill)
3. describe models of effective cross-cultural communication, assessment, and physician–patient negotiation and identify common challenges in cross-cultural communication (for example, trust, style) (Objective 22 – knowledge)
4. assess and enhance patient adherence based on the patient's explanatory model. Describe ways to enhance patient adherence by collaborating with traditional and other community healers (Objective 25 – knowledge, skill).

Instructional Materials
Presentation assignment and guidelines, distributed some weeks prior to the presentation date to learners who will be presenting cases; materials requested by residents/students to facilitate case presentations; session objectives; commitment to change forms.

Time Schedule
00:00 – 00:03   Session introduction
00:03 – 00:45   Case presentation (maximum of seven six-minute case presentations)
00:45 – 00:55   Group discussion of common themes and session conclusion
00:55 – 01:00   Portfolio and commitment to change

Process
Distribute presentation assignment and guidelines (*see* below) some weeks prior to the presentation date to learners who have been assigned to present cases. Instructors may want to review proposed cases with learners prior to the presentation date for appropriateness and relevance.
1. Introduction (3 minutes): this session requires only a brief introduction to present the session objectives to the learners, and explain how this session is part of the larger culturally responsive care curriculum.
2. Case presentations (42 minutes): each learner presents a case example of their work with a patient that illustrates culturally responsive care in terms of negotiating a culturally responsive treatment plan, incorporation of patient's health beliefs in the treatment plan, as well as collaboration with alternative or ethno-medical healers. Relevant health outcomes should be mentioned.

3. Group discussion of common themes and session conclusion (10 minutes): use facilitation to engage all learners in discussion. Invite learners to identify any commonalities they observed in the case presentations in terms of clinical challenges and positive interventions.

4. Portfolio (5 minutes): learners who presented cases should add them to their portfolios. All learners have the opportunity to write about new insights and knowledge gained from the case presentations (listening to others, and for second year residents, preparing their own presentations). Encourage learners to make at least one commitment to change based on today's session and place the form in their portfolios.

Cautionary Note

Once learners begin this project, they will be challenged to keep their presentation brief and focused on the cultural aspects of the case. They may require guidance in pulling together relevant data instead of potentially presenting typical history and physical data, which may not be relevant to the task at hand.

Instructor Note

This exercise could easily be expanded into 30 minutes per learner, if time permits in your curriculum. Each learner presentation would be 20 minutes with 10 minutes for discussion. The presentation outline might be as follows: 1. case presentation; 2. formal discussion of the health belief system held by the patient; 3. a brief description of the cross-cultural communication model used by the resident; and 4. personal insights gained by the resident in the exploration of the case. Learners might use a PowerPoint presentation format to share their information with the group. Each presentation would be followed by discussion. The other learners should complete a formal evaluation of each of these presentations to assist the presenter in honing presentation skills.

Resources

Aberegg SK, Terry PB. Medical decision-making and healthcare disparities: The physician's role. *J Lab Clin Med*. 2004 Jul; **144**(1): 11–17.

Balsa AI, Seiler N, McGuire TG, *et al*. Clinical uncertainty and healthcare disparities. *Am J Law Med*. 2003; **29**(2–3): 203–19.

Lewis-Fernandez R, Diaz, N. The cultural formulation: a method for assessing cultural factors affecting the clinical encounter. *Psychiatr Q*. 2002; **73**(4): 271–95.

Lu FG, Lim R, Mezzich JE. Issues in the assessment and diagnosis of culturally diverse individuals. In: Oldham J, Riba M, editors. *Review of Psychiatry*, vol. 14. Washington, DC: American Psychiatric Press; 1995. pp. 477–510.

Thiel de Bocanegra H, Gany F. Good provider, good patient: changing behaviors to eliminate disparities in healthcare. *Am J Manag Care*. 2004 Sep; **10** Spec No: SP20–8.

SESSION 29 – RESIDENT HANDOUT Cultural Medicine Case Presentation Preparation Guidelines

You are to prepare a six-minute presentation of a case that illustrates your culturally responsive work with a patient. The presentation will be on (insert date here), and you will be one of (insert number) presenters that day.

Objectives

The objectives of these presentations are to:

1. describe the patient's historical model of health belief (if applicable) and the questions about health practices and beliefs that were important to your understanding of that patient's model
2. identify healing traditions and beliefs of your patient and/or their family, including ethno-medical beliefs and use of ethno-medical healers.
3. describe any model of cross-cultural communication, assessment, and clinician–patient negotiation that you used and identify any challenges you faced (for example, trust, style).
4. if appropriate, describe how you worked to enhance patient adherence by collaborating with traditional and other community healers.

Instructions

1. Select a case where a health belief of the patient was relevant to your care. You should be able to discuss the health belief in the context of any relevant historical model of health care belief. In selecting your case pick one where negotiation of a care plan that incorporated the patient's health beliefs was important and/or where collaboration with alternative or ethno-medical healers took place.
2. You may discuss your case selection with the course instructor in terms of appropriateness and relevance of the case to the cultural medicine curriculum and session goals.
3. Given the brief time allotted for the presentation, be very judicious in selecting which aspects of the case to include. For example, share only case history data that directly applies to the health belief in question, use of alternative/complementary medicine and any cultural negotiation of the treatment plan.
4. Be sure to share insights you have gained about the health belief in question from research you did on that belief.
5. Practice your presentation – six minutes is brief, timing is important.

SESSION 30 Annual Review of Individual Cultural Competency Commitments

Session Description

The final session in each year of the three-year curriculum (sessions 10, 20, and 30) provides an opportunity for each learner to use reflection and self-assessment to reflect upon their portfolio entries and their progress to date. Learners will be provided with the opportunity to share with each other, if they choose to, some of their areas of positive growth, as well as remaining challenges. There will also be time for general discussion in relation to ways for reducing bias of the providers and for addressing disparities for patients within their practice environment. The group might select one thing to work on over the next academic year. In the second and third year, the group should spend some time in this session discussing progress over the past year on their target goal.

Session Objectives

After participation in the session, learners should be better able to:
1. become aware of their own cultural heritage, gender, class, ethnic-racial identity, sexual orientation, disability, age and spirituality; be able to reflect on it and describe it (Objective 2 – awareness, skill)
2. recognize their own potential for bias and stereotyping, be able to identify their own stereotypes and biases and explore how their attitudes, biases and stereotypes affect clinical encounters, clinical decision-making and quality of care (Objective 12 – awareness, knowledge)
3. describe strategies for reducing physician's own biases, and those of others and demonstrate strategies to assess, manage, and reduce bias and its effects in the clinical encounter and in clinical practice (Objective 15 – skill)
4. describe patterns of health care disparities that can result, at least in part, from clinician bias, recognize disparities that are amenable to intervention, and value eliminating disparities (Objective 20 – attitude, knowledge).

Instructional Materials

Flip chart and pens; the entire set of objectives for the Cultural Competence Curriculum for review; collected learner materials for each learner (presentations, quizzes, reflective writings, commitments to change, etc.), these should be distributed to each learner at the start of the session.

Time Schedule

00:00 – 00:05 Session introduction
00:05 – 00:20 Independent review of portfolio including the commitments to change
00:20 – 00:40 Open discussion
00:40 – 00:55 Plan for change, think-pair-share
00:55 – 01:00 Session conclusion

Process

1. Introduction (5 minutes): this session requires only a brief introduction to the importance of this session as part of the larger culturally responsive care curriculum.
2. Independent review (15 minutes): learners are provided with their portfolio of materials collected over the course of their participation in the cultural medicine curriculum (including orientation materials for first year residents). Ask them to review the materials with an eye to their positive growth, areas for further and future growth, the degree to which they have been able to fulfill their commitments, and any barriers faced in fulfilling those commitments. Learners may wish to highlight outstanding learning experiences and/or clinical encounters over the past year.
3. Open discussion (20 minutes): here the group is invited to share their findings from the independent review. Successes, frustrations, and barriers can be highlighted by the group

facilitator on flip charts at the front of the room. A revisiting of the Cultural Curriculum Objectives can be helpful and included as part of this discussion. The skills of facilitation will help ensure a student-centered discussion.

4. Personal goals/think-pair-share (15 minutes): looking to the future, learners are asked to write their personal goals for professional growth toward culturally responsive care, including any personal areas of bias, stereotyping and/or discomfort. Next, each learner shares these with a partner, and finally the group as a whole joins a larger discussion of future learning goals.

5. Session conclusion (5 minutes): first, this is an opportunity to thank the learners for their input today and over this segment of the curriculum (Sessions A, B, C and 21–30). Second, commend the seniors for their accomplishment in completing the 33-session curriculum. Remind them that they will need to complete and return any post-participation materials. Third, remind the returning students that the curriculum uses a spiral model. In the next year, the returning learners will revisit each of the six units in Sessions 1–10 of the curriculum. Collect all portfolios at the end of the session.

Instructor Note

Learners often have a tendency to focus more on the negative than the positive in their own professional trajectory. It is important that the facilitator help learners share observed areas of growth and accomplishment in a balanced fashion with frustrations/challenges. For the seniors, this should be more of a celebration than an evaluation.

Resources

Betancourt JR. Cultural competence and medical education: many names, many perspectives, one goal. *Acad Med.* 2006 Jun; **81**(6): 499–501.

Chambers N. Close encounters: the use of critical reflective analysis as an evaluation tool in teaching and learning. *J Adv Nurs.* 1999; **29**(4): 950–7.

Like RC. Culturally competent family medicine: transforming clinical practice and ourselves. *Am Fam Physician.* 2005 Dec; **72**(11): 2189.

Murray-Garcia JL, Harrell S, Garcia JA, *et al.* Self-reflection in multicultural training: be careful what you ask for. *Acad Med.* 2005 Jul; **80**(7): 694–701.

Section 4

Teaching Techniques

Teaching Techniques:
Overview and Table of Contents

The teaching techniques described in this section are divided into five categories.

Attention Grabbers

TEACHING TECHNIQUE 1 Brainstorming and Best-Worst Warm-Up

Description

With brainstorming, the instructor engages the group in an open exchange of information generally to make a list of issues or possible solutions in relation to a topic under discussion. It is designed to allow a group of people to creatively generate a large number of ideas related to a specific topic by creating a process that is free of criticism and judgment. This method can also be used to bring a team together to think about a given problem or challenge and to generate solutions. The intent is to get all solutions 'out on the table', rather than to develop a particular solution, or to select the best solution. The best-worst warm-up is a variant used typically as an opener, a way to capture learners' attention at the beginning of a session by exploring the polarities.

Uses

❏ Brainstorming is used to encourage learners to think broadly about possible issues or problem solutions in relation to issues like access, quality of care, or community health challenges. The objective is to generate many ideas in relation to addressing a challenge.

❏ The best-worst warm-up can be used to gather needs assessment information on a topic of interest (i.e. gaps in learner awareness, knowledge, attitude, or perceived skills); to introduce a session or topic; as a lead-in to the session objectives; or to open up a new discussion and build learner interest in the topic.

Process

Structured Brainstorming

There are several rules to follow when conducting a structured brainstorming session.

1. Identify the topic to be discussed or the problem to be solved and seek group agreement. Without such agreement, it is easy to digress and be unproductive.
2. Each person expresses ideas in turn. No criticism is to be allowed.
3. Write down ideas as they are expressed. Ideas should not be interpreted or analyzed during a brainstorming session.
4. Keep going around the room and adding ideas until each person has 'passed'.
5. Review the list and discard any duplicates. In this process all ideas are recognized. An open dialogue should be promoted by acknowledging each member's contribution equally.

Unstructured Brainstorming

Unstructured brainstorming differs only in the way ideas are generated. There is free discussion with learners calling out answers until all ideas get put on paper. Brainstorming can also be done silently (no spoken words) with each person taking turns adding ideas to a growing written list. This last approach is a powerful way for a group to summarize what it has learned in a given curriculum or to build a list of concerns or needs.

Best-Worst Warm-Up

Divide the group into small groups (no more than six people in each). Instruct half of the groups to construct the positive list (e.g. best, proudest, strengths) and the other half to compose the negative lists (e.g. worst, most embarrassing, weaknesses, barriers). Give the groups about five minutes to make their lists – monitor the groups and shorten or extend the time as required. The facilitator then guides the groups through reporting and making a single list. A flip chart with a line drawn down the middle and a single word (positive or negative) at the top of each column is sufficient to record the groups' lists. The facilitator should prepare a master list including the most important positives and negatives. This can be used during the discussion to ensure that all of the important items are included. Refer to debriefing (Technique 15) for hints on guiding the discussion.

Time Required

Generally about 10–20 minutes, depending on complexity of topic and specific method used.

Group Size and Structure

Structured brainstorming is best suited to small groups (no more than 25); unstructured brainstorming and the best-worst warm-up can be successful even with large groups of students although they might be more effective if coupled with think-write-share.

Materials

May use electronic means (e.g. computer with projector, overhead projector), flip chart, or white board to record the lists generated by the group.

Advantages

Unstructured brainstorming and best-worst warm-up can be quick and easy methods to engage learners in a topic. They can help generate learner interest and assess learner needs at the beginning of a session. The structured method is a powerful way for a group to address potential solutions to identified issues, challenges, or problems.

Limitations

The structured method takes more time, but tends to ensure that all participate. In contrast, the unstructured method takes less time, but does not ensure full participation in the discussion.

Resources

Geuna S, Giacobini-Robecchi MG. The use of brainstorming for teaching human anatomy. *Anat Rec.* 2002 Oct 15; **269**(5): 214–6.

Munoz Adanez A. Does quantity generate quality? Testing the fundamental principle of brainstorming. *Span J Psychol.* 2005 Nov; **8**(2): 215–20.

Schweinfurth JM. Interactive instruction in otolaryngology resident education. *Otolaryngol Clin North Am.* 2007 Dec; **40**(6): 1203–14, vi.

TEACHING TECHNIQUE 2 Openers and Closers

Description
The opening and closing moments crucial to success of a session. The opening sets the tone for the entire session, gains the learners' attention, and places the session into context. The session introduction can be enhanced with an appropriate opener as opposed to (or in addition to) the standard opening of a recitation of the session objectives. At times you want to 'grab' your learners' attention with a higher impact opening. The final moments of a teaching/learning session can help ensure that the learners have gained key learning points and add to the impact of the session.

Uses
Openers are used to gain the learners' attention and focus them on the session topic and to start a session on a strong positive note. Closers ensure that learners gain the important take home points and can help learners integrate information and apply it later.

Opener Process
1. Select an appropriate type of opener. Some options include: present the agenda; use a visual (chart, photo, model, slide, cartoon); ask a question (rhetorical or interactive); use a dramatic action (e.g. a loud noise, or surprise interaction between the speakers); use a quotation; present a fact or statistic to demonstrate the importance of the topic; tell a joke or funny story; tell a personal anecdote; appeal directly to the learners' self-interest.
2. Select the source material and purchase it and/or obtain permission to show the material in your session, if required.
3. Practice using the opener to make sure your delivery is optimal. Delivery matters.

Closer Process
1. Identify the key take-home points. Plan the closer for impact.
2. Select closer. It can list take-home points, repeat objectives, direct learners to resources or other study materials, tie the content to a past session or overall curriculum, provide an application assignment, or attempt to inspire learners to make changes in their practice behaviors. A summary image (e.g. chart, graph, illustration) can be very powerful.
3. Use of commitment to change can enhance this process.

Time Required
Maximum of three minutes for each. Many take only one minute.

Group Size and Structure
Any size group.

Materials
Copy of the stimulus material for opener and concisely written closer.

Advantages
Varying your opening in a multi-session curriculum helps keep the learners interested and attentive. Learners remember best what they hear last, so the closer can help enhance impact with a strong take-home message. This time can also be used to gain a commitment from learners as to how they will take the 'lesson' and apply it in the workplace.

Limitations
Both the opener and closer should fit the subject and objectives for the session. Just like openers, closers should be varied in a multi-session program to maintain impact.

Cautionary Note
Be careful with the use of jokes. It is ill advised to use a joke that makes fun of ANY group of people. Personal anecdotes tend to be better received (but must relate to objectives).

Resource
Anderson JB. *Speaking to Groups: Eyeball to eyeball*. Vienna, VA: Windmoor Press; 1989.

TEACHING TECHNIQUE 3 Video Clips

Description

A video clip is a short excerpt of video, generally selected from a longer video production (television program, movie, educational media). The video clip, sometimes called a 'trigger film/tape', should be selected to meet a specific curricular objective. Teachers can rarely afford the time to show a longer video simply to entertain learners. In one-hour teaching sessions like those in this curriculum, it is recommended that you carefully select a portion of five minutes or less to stimulate discussion related to a specific concept, and of no more than 10 minutes at a time, for any purpose.

Many video resources are available and specifically designed to enhance cultural competence education. Some of these include already prepared short clips; however, many are longer presentations or include longer video clips of 10–30 minutes. These should be excerpted prior to showing or used with planned pauses for discussion.

Uses

❑ To introduce a topic or concept with high impact – video is more powerful than words.
❑ To provide a positive or negative example of an interpersonal or communication skill.
❑ To prompt discussion in relation to a specific curricular topic or learner outcome objective.

Process

1. Determine that a video clip is the optimal method for your purpose. Plan the teaching session and then select the clip.
2. Select the source material and purchase it and/or obtain permission to show the material in your session.
3. Select the specific brief clip and prepare it for showing – it may need to be 'captured' or 'copied' and placed on a computer or burned onto a DVD. This is particularly true if more than one clip is to be used in a single session. Never use a clip that you have not previewed, no matter how good the description sounds or how compelling the recommendations from colleagues. Remember to limit the clip to the relevant section only.
4. Check to make sure that a) the equipment is available and works; b) your video clip can be seen and heard in the room to be used; and c) the video/DVD is cued to the correct point if viewing from the original.
5. Introduce the clip. You may need to provide a description of the story plot if the clip is taken from a movie, television program, or extended video. Provide the learners with a challenge, for example:
   - Imagine that you are the provider in this clip; what would you do next and why?
   - As you watch this video clip, try to identify the ethical challenge facing the provider and patient.
   - While watching this clip, make note of the questions you have in regard to this patient's health belief system.
   - As you watch the video, note any feelings that are triggered in you by the interactions.
6. Make sure that the purpose for using the clip is clear and that an activity follows that meets the session objective. Repeat the challenge after the video clip is shown, to lead into the planned activity.
7. Use the skills of 'facilitation' and 'debriefing' to extend the impact of the segment or session that follows use of the video clip.

Time Required

With a three-minute clip, the time required for viewing and discussion would generally be less than 10 minutes.

Group Size and Structure

Any size group is acceptable. With very large groups, the clip could be followed by think-write-share or think-pair-share to stimulate broader discussion.

Materials

Original video materials (purchased or with permission to use obtained); video clip; and projection set-up.

Advantages

Short video clips grab an audience's attention and can prompt relevant discussion; short video clips (five minutes or less) provide the benefits of a longer video without excess expenditure of valuable session time; pictures can have a greater impact and can be remembered for longer than discussion alone.

Limitations

The selected clip must address the concept of interest; must be at the level of the learners; must be long enough to get the point across and short enough to maintain focus on the relevant issues.

Cautionary Notes

1. Use video clips sparingly within the cultural competence curriculum to maximize their impact.
2. When using video for projection on a large screen (e.g. in an auditorium) ensure that the quality of both video (pixels) and audio (volume without distortion) are sufficient for viewing.

Resources

Alexander M, Hall MN, Pettice YJ. Cinemeducation: an innovative approach to teaching psychosocial medical care. *Fam Med*. 1994; **26**(7): 430–3.

Alexander M, Lenahan P, Pavlov A. *Cinemeducation: A comprehensive guide to using film in medical education.* Oxford: Radcliffe; 2004.

Azer SA. Twelve tips for creating trigger images for problem-based learning cases. *Med Teach*. 2007 Mar; **29**(2–3): 93–7.

Ber R, Alroy G. Teaching professionalism with the aid of trigger films. *Med Teach*. 2002; **24**(5): 528–31.

Ber R, Alroy G. Twenty years of experience using trigger films as a teaching tool. *Acad Med*. 2001 Jun; **76**(6): 656–8.

Rabinowitz D, Melzer-Geva M, Ber R. Teaching the cultural dimensions of the patient-physician relationship: a novel approach using didactic trigger films. *Med Teach*. 2002 Mar; **24**(2): 181–5.

Skill Builders

TEACHING TECHNIQUE 4 Expanded Cases and Conferences

Description

With this technique the instructor takes advantage of existing case presentation/discussion opportunities to infuse these occasions with relevant additional content in relation to cultural competence.

Uses

❏ To integrate issues of cultural competence into standard clinical case discussion.
❏ To infuse classroom and clinical settings with relevant discussions in relation to issues of health care disparities, cultural competence, and patient-centered care.

Process

1. Review conference or didactic curriculum schedule to consider opportunities to infuse cultural competence into the curriculum.
2. Discuss this as a program goal with other faculty members.
3. Work with faculty to refine the cultural competence curriculum objectives to meet your program's goals.
4. Have cultural questions available for presenters and encourage them to incorporate these into their case presentations, didactic presentations and research article reviews, as appropriate.
5. Be a role model in your teaching.

Time Required

One to 20 minutes per case depending on the focus.

Group Size and Structure

Any size group.

Materials

Lists of relevant questions that can be used to expand discussion. Attached are three sets of questions directly related to the objectives of this curriculum: a) related to specific patient cases; b) related to topical presentation; and c) related to discussions of research articles.

Advantage

Takes advantage of existing common teaching practice, the use of cases and case presentations.

Limitation

Should not be used with every case, nor in every case-based session; the questions should be kept ready for an occasion when their use might add to the discussion or enhance care for the patient (or case) under discussion, or for future patients.

Questions Related to Specific Patient Cases

Objectives	Questions for Cases
8. Identify healing traditions and beliefs of patients and/or their families, including ethno-medical beliefs. Ask questions in a non-judgmental manner to elicit patient preferences, listen and respond appropriately to patient feedback about key cross-cultural issues. Elicit additional information about ethno-medical conditions and ethno-medical healers.	Any role for alternative or complementary medicine for this patient? Could it help or have helped? Did it hinder?
12. Recognize their own potential for bias and stereotyping, be able to identify their own stereotypes and biases and explore how their attitudes, biases and stereotypes affect clinical encounters, clinical decision-making and quality of care.	Have the attitudes, biases or stereotypes of providers (related to appearance, race, ethnicity, economic status, sex, sexual preference, religion, culture, etc.) affected care and/or outcomes for this patient? If yes, how?
15. Describe strategies for reducing physician's own biases, and those of others, and demonstrate strategies to assess, manage, and reduce bias and its effects in the clinical encounter and in clinical practice.	How can we reduce the impact of any biases in the care of future patients?
17. Recognize and describe how access, historical, political, environmental, and institutional factors (including racism and discrimination) impact health and underlie health and health care disparities.	Were any health care disparities already affecting the patient's health status prior to us seeing the patient? How can we avoid health disparities for future patients?
18. Identify how race, ethnicity and social determinants of health (e.g. education, culture, socioeconomic status, housing, and employment) affect health and health care quality, cost, and outcomes.	Any concerns about the patient's ability or willingness to adhere to the treatment plan, and how did this play a role in outcomes?
20. Describe patterns of health care disparities that can result, at least in part, from clinician bias, recognize disparities that are amenable to intervention and value eliminating disparities.	What action can we take to help eliminate any disparity affecting this patient?
21. Describe systemic and medical-encounter issues related to health care disparities, including communication issues, clinical decision-making, and patient preferences.	Any discrepancies between the assessment and plan, and the patient's health belief system? Anything omitted from the plan based on 'who' this patient is (e.g. likeable, deserving, living circumstances) or based on patient preferences? Consequences?
22. Describe models of effective cross-cultural communication, assessment, and physician–patient negotiation and identify common challenges in cross-cultural communication (e.g. trust).	Were there communication challenges in the care of this patient? If so, how were they addressed and what was the impact on care and outcomes?
25. Assess and enhance patient adherence based on the patient's explanatory model. Describe ways to enhance patient adherence by collaborating with traditional and other community healers.	If patient adherence was an issue, what might we do to enhance it? How might additional negotiation help?

Questions Related to Topical Presentations

Objectives	Topic-Related Questions
4. Identify patterns of national data on health, health care disparities, and quality of health care, and be able to discuss.	What patterns of disparities have been identified in relation to this topic/medical problem?
5. Discuss the epidemiology of health and health care disparities for the local community using *Healthy People 2010* and other resources.	Related to this topic/medical problem, what health care disparities exist locally, in the county, state or nation? How are we doing in addressing them for our patients?
6. Value the importance of social determinants and community factors on health and strive to address them.	In relation to the topic, which social determinants in our community that contribute to disparities and how can we address them?
7. Describe historical models of common health beliefs (for example, illness in the context of 'hot and cold'), and identify questions about health practices and beliefs that might be important in a specific local community.	Are there any common health beliefs or practices in our community related to this topic/medical problem? How should we address them?

Objectives	Topic-Related Questions
8. Identify healing traditions and beliefs of patients and/or their families, including ethno-medical beliefs. Ask questions in a non-judgmental manner to elicit patient preferences, listen and respond appropriately to patient feedback about key cross-cultural issues. Elicit additional information about ethno-medical conditions and ethno-medical healers.	What role do alternative or ethno-medical healers play in our community in relation to this topic/medical problem? How should we be addressing this in our care plans?

Questions Related to Research Articles and Presentations of Literature

Objectives	Literature-Related Questions
3. Value the importance of diversity in health care and address the challenges and opportunities it poses.	Who were the participants in the study? How were they selected? How well did they reflect the demographics of our patient population?
7. Describe historical models of common health beliefs (for example, illness in the context of 'hot and cold'), and identify questions about health practices and beliefs that might be important in a specific local community.	How were the health beliefs and cultural context of patients taken into consideration in this study? What more could have been done?
19. Identify and discuss key areas of disparities described in *Healthy People 2010* and the Institute of Medicine's Report, *Unequal Treatment* and discuss barriers to eliminating health disparities.	Was the issue of health care disparities addressed in the article? Should it have been? Why or why not?
26. Critically appraise the literature as it relates to health disparities, including systems issues and quality in health care.	How will the results of the study impact health care disparities – improve, make worse, no impact? Why?

Resources

Betancourt JR, Green AR, Carrillo JE, *et al*. Defining cultural competence: a practical framework for addressing racial/ethnic disparities in health and health care. *Pub Health Rep*. 2003; **118**(4): 293–302.

Campinha-Bacote J. *The Process of Cultural Competence in the Delivery of Health Care Services: A culturally competent model of care*. 3rd ed. Cincinnati, OH: Transcultural CARE Associates; 1999.

Carrillo JE, Green AR, Betancourt JR. Cross-cultural primary care: a patient-based approach. *Ann Intern Med*. 1999; **130**(10): 829–34.

Kleinman A, Eisenberg L, Good B. Culture, illness, and care: clinical lessons from anthropologic and cross-cultural research. *Ann Intern Med*. 1978; **88**: 251–8.

National Standards for Culturally and Linguistically Appropriate Services in Health Care: Final Report. Rockville, MD: US Department of Health and Human Services, Office of Minority Health; 2001 Mar.

Purnell L. The Purnell Model for cultural competence. *J Transcult Nurs*. 2002; **13**(3): 193–6.

Smedley BD, Stith AY, Nelson AR, editors. IOM Report: *Unequal Treatment: Confronting Racial and Ethnic Disparities in Health Care*. Board on Health Sciences Policy. Washington, DC: National Academies Press; 2002. Available from: http://www.iom.edu/CMS/3740/4475.aspx

TEACHING TECHNIQUE 5 Formal Presentation (Lecture and Demonstration)

Description
With this method, the presenter makes an oral presentation of information, often using visual aids, and the learner listens and may take notes. The formal presentation method typically uses a one-way channel of communication, from instructor to learner. Types of formal presentations include lectures, symposia, panel presentations, and demonstrations. Demonstrations are often used as an initial introduction to specific techniques in the areas of interpersonal skills, clinical skills, and technical skills. Demonstrations help learners gain knowledge about 'how to' do something.

Use
To promote acquisition of knowledge.

Process
Formal presentations play an important role in many teaching sessions lasting one hour or more. It is important to keep these presentations short – generally no more than 10–20 minutes per lecture or demonstration. Each presentation should include the standard three parts: introduction, body, and conclusion. *See* the section on openers and closers (Technique 2) for some hints on ways to grab the learners' attention and ensure impact. Interaction is encouraged with formal presentations. Techniques like progressive disclosure cases, video clips with debriefing, quizzes, and think-write-share, can extend the impact of formal presentations and aid the integration of learner-centered activities into large group teaching/learning sessions.

Time Required
Variable, recommended lecturing no more than 10–20 minutes without integration of other techniques.

Group Size and Structure
Any size, although generally mid-sized to very large groups.

Materials
Visual aids.

Advantages
Instructors can present substantial amounts of information in a short period of time, and introduce the relevant knowledge to support all other competencies. Formal presentations can provide new and otherwise inaccessible material, and may be used to stimulate learner interest in further study. May be recorded for future use and can accommodate a large number of participants.

Limitations
The formal presentation is a passive learning modality, providing little chance for independent thinking. Presenters must be wary of positioning the content at their own level of understanding rather than that of the learners. It can be difficult to assess degree of impact on individual learners. Lectures have limited effectiveness in teaching anything other than knowledge.

Resources
Collins J. Education techniques for lifelong learning: giving a PowerPoint presentation: the art of communicating effectively. *Radiographics*. 2004 Jul–Aug; **24**(4): 1185–92.

Selby G, Walker V, Diwakar V. A comparison of teaching methods: interactive lecture versus game playing. *Med Teach*. 2007 Nov; **29**(9): 972–4.

■ CURRICULUM FOR CULTURALLY RESPONSIVE HEALTH CARE

TEACHING TECHNIQUE 6 Independent Study Using Written or Technology-Based Materials

Description

Independent study activities are typically designed to enhance and support other instructional activities. The assignment or activity is generally accomplished entirely by the individual learner (or group of learners), usually using resource materials, e.g. readings, internet resources, computer-assisted instructional packages, online databases, video/audio recording, etc. Materials may be learner selected or teacher selected. Tasks also often include completion of summaries, reflections, questions, narratives, cases or quizzes.

Uses

Independent activities can be used to promote awareness, independent learning, increased knowledge, and improved problem solving.

Process

The instructor should carefully choose activities to ensure that they are relevant to immediate learner outcome objectives (*see* Section 7 for ideas). If materials are to be learner selected, the instructor should provide guidance in the form of recommended references or resource listings. If materials are to be instructor selected, either provide the materials (hard copy/electronic reserve) or provide the specific references and how to locate each.

It is very important to integrate these materials into classroom activities. Assign only materials that you will use, and attempt to use them in a way that makes completion of the independent assignment important to the goals of the session. Apply the materials in the session (e.g. use as a stimulus for initial discussion), or build on the materials, as opposed to reviewing the content of the materials during the session. Failure to do these things will generally result in learners' failure to complete future independent activities.

Example Methods for Integration

❏ Awareness – learners are asked to come to class prepared to discuss the personal impact of the independent material.
❏ Knowledge/problem solving – instructors could introduce a case study that requires immediate application of knowledge; instructors may engage learners in a game or audience response system quiz or poll to assess learning at the beginning of the session.
❏ Communication skills/professionalism – the instructor can begin the session with an exercise like best-worst warm-up or brainstorming to have the group immediately use information in the readings; instructor might open the session with a narrative writing exercise based on the materials reviewed or completed prior to class.

Time Required

Variable depending on the assignment – generally no more than one or two hours for an independent study assignment prior to a session.

Group Size and Structure

Any size group.

Materials

A wide variety of materials including text materials, e-materials or activities, self-study modules (paper or electronic), etc. may be used.

Advantages

Independent study fosters independent learning skills. The learner can progress at his/her own rate, which enriches presentations and other learning experiences. Learners can gain the prerequisite knowledge for all other areas of competence. Computers are widely available, with many online resources typically available at most university sites.

Limitations

Learners must complete their independent assignments for this technique to be effective – completion of a brief product (summary of chapter, review form for article critique, reflection on web-based activity) often enhances compliance with the independent activity. Many articles and books are only partially relevant to immediate objectives, so materials must be carefully selected. Beware that it may be hard to locate materials at learners' level, and that audio-visual or computer-based materials are time consuming and expensive to develop.

Resources

McKimm J, Jollie C, Cantillon P. ABC's of teaching and learning: web based learning. *BMJ*. 2003; **326**(7394): 870–3.

Wendler MC, Struthers R. Bridging culture on-line: strategies for teaching cultural sensitivity. *J Prof Nurs*. 2002 Nov–Dec; **18**(6): 320–7.

TEACHING TECHNIQUE 7 Role Play

Description
Role play as a teaching strategy is typically implemented early in an instructional process to help learners acquire interpersonal and communication skills through guided practice. Two types of role play can be used – classic role play and oral simulation of practitioner–patient interaction. Each is described separately below.

CLASSIC ROLE PLAY
In use of classic role play, each participant temporarily adopts a specified role and tries to behave in ways characteristic of a person in that role. Role playing can be incorporated into small group teaching or used for demonstration purposes for a large group. Learners work in groups of three, each taking a role (e.g. patient, interviewer, observer).

Uses
This is a low-risk method for learners to practice new interaction skills before using them with patients.

Process
1. Prepare all materials in advance. You will need instructions for each role – patient (three cases, keeping details as simple as possible), provider/interviewer (same for all cases) and the observer (same for all cases). Sessions that include role play are generally best done with a team of at least two instructors.
2. The session typically begins with an introduction to the concept and often includes a demonstration of the required role play conducted by the instructors.
3. Divide the group into role play subgroups of three learners each. Provide clear instructions to the learners about the activity:
   a) exactly how much time for each round (generally 5–10 minutes per round);
   b) how to divide the time between the 'interview' and the feedback; and
   c) instructions for the feedback – 'interviewer' speaks first on what went well and what he/she would have done differently, 'patient' next with brief balanced positive and constructive feedback, and then the 'observer' provides feedback on the interaction and/ or on the content (as instructed).
4. Conduct the actual role play, overseeing the process carefully to insure that all groups are staying on task.
5. Debrief the activity. Be prepared to handle the skeptics as well as any unexpected insights.

Time Required
Depends on the task and the number of 'rounds'. Typically there are three rounds, to allow each learner to play the patient, the interviewer, and the observer. The rounds rarely last more than 5–10 minutes. If time is very limited, it is permissible to use two rounds, using pairs (interviewer and patient, with no observer).

Group Size and Structure
Typically done in a workshop setting with no more than 20–30 learners.

Materials
Separate directions and scripts for each role – patient, interviewer and observer; and three sets of patient information, one for each round, each of which includes circumstances, tone, and answers to key expected questions.

Advantages
Role play encourages active participation, and can be used when 'real' experiences are not readily available. It can provide practice before the learner tries out the skills on patients, and learners may develop insights about human feelings and relations. This technique can also be

used to help residents learn how to provide feedback, using a student for one role, or to work in collaborative teams, using other health care providers for roles.

Limitations
Learning objectives and tasks must be clearly outlined in order to maintain learner focus and prevent task degeneration. Role play depends heavily on the learner's imagination and willingness to participate, and can have unpredictable outcomes, so debriefing is very important.

ORAL SIMULATION OF PRACTITIONER–PATIENT INTERACTION (Instructor-Controlled and Instructor-Dependent)

Description
This technique begins with the learner being provided with a basic clinical scenario. The instructor (or standardized patient) then begins to play the role of a patient or family member, with the learner's task to gain (or provide) appropriate information at a specific point in the care process.

Uses
This method can be used to enhance interaction skills, and to teach interviewing of difficult patients or in sensitive areas, to provide counseling, or to provide patient education. It is a technique often used in Introduction to Clinical Medicine or Doctoring courses, and in cultural competence training at all levels.

Process
Instructor as Actor:
1. Begins with the group being provided with a basic clinical scenario and a task. Example – a homeless teenager comes to clinic complaining of a discharge from penis. Task for group is to conduct a culturally sensitive interview and to gather medical data, but also to gather C-HEADDSS data (culture, home, education, activities, drugs, depression, sex, suicide).[1]
2. Progressive interview using time-in/time-out – the learners will take turns acting as the interviewer. The learner can call time-out to ask for advice from the other students. The instructor can call time-out (making a 'T' with his/her two hands) to make a point or to change interviewer. The interview generally moves fairly quickly, no more than a couple of minutes per learner.
3. After each learner has had an opportunity to interview the instructor/patient, the instructor leads a discussion of the process and the main learning points. Learners may provide feedback to each other.

Standardized Patient (SP): the process is the same except for the discussion. With an SP, the interview may last much longer, with conversations among the students at key time-out points in terms of what should be asked and how it should be asked. The group may provide feedback to each learner at the end of their turn or the SP may provide feedback to each person at the end of the interview. Rules need to be established in terms of who can call a time-out. Generally, only the current interviewer or the instructor can call a time-out. During a time-out the SP bows his/her head and is 'not in the room'. When time-in is called then the patient returns to the point in the interview where the time-out was called with no apparent interruption in the interview.

Time Required
Depends on purpose of simulation, generally no more than 20 minutes per encounter.

Group Size and Structure
Small group with instructor (5–8 learners).

Materials
Case scenario (in format of SP case), task for learners, SP if possible.

Advantages
Oral simulation can ensure participation of all learners, and can be used when 'real' experiences

are not readily available. It can provide practice before the learner tries out the skills on patients, and learners may develop insights about human feelings and relations.

Limitations

Instructor dependent, requires skilled facilitation, and if taking dual role (instructor/actor) requires intense focus and multi-tasking abilities. Reflection and commitment to change can be used to expand impact of either technique.

Reference

1. Cohen E, Mackenzie RG, Yates GL. HEADSS, a psychosocial risk assessment instrument: implications for designing effective intervention programs for runaway youth. *J Adolesc Health*. 1991 Nov; **12**(7): 539–44.

Resources

Christiaens G, Baldwin JH. Use of dyadic role playing to increase student participation. *Nurse Educator*. 2002; **27**(6): 251–4.

Joyner B, Young L. Teaching medical students using role play: twelve tips for successful role plays. *Med Teach*. 2006 May; **28**(3): 225–9.

Shearer R, Davidhizar R. Using role play to develop cultural competence. *J Nurs Educ*. 2003 Jun; **42**(6): 273–6.

Stafford F. The significance of de-roling and debriefing in training medical students using simulation to train medical students. *Med Educat*. 2005 Nov; **39**(11): 1083–5.

TEACHING TECHNIQUE 8 Standardized Patients

Description

Standardized patients (SPs) can be a useful addition to an instructional program, particularly in the teaching of interviewing, counseling, and interpersonal skills. SPs are actors trained to portray a specific patient role in a consistent and accurate manner. They are trained to interact as the original patient would and to react differentially depending on how the health professional interacts with them, as well as depending upon what the health professional asks. Research has shown that SPs, when appropriately trained, can perform complicated cases, even those involving simulated physical findings in a realistic and reliable manner. SPs can also be trained to assess learners and to provide appropriate feedback.

Uses

SPs can be used in the classroom as adjunct to formal presentations when skills are demonstrated or within group interviews as a stimulus for group discussion on clinical issues. However, the primary strength of the technique is in one-to-one interviews between the patient and the health professional. In this context, the technique provides a standardized clinical stimulus for all learners and has the unique advantage of allowing for patient feedback to the learner.

Process

1. Develop an SP case or select one from those your local medical school already has prepared (case development protocol attached).
2. Develop rating tools and/or instructions for the specific usage.
3. Integrate use of the SP into the teaching situation (demonstration, oral simulation, one-to-one teaching).
4. Provide feedback where appropriate – for one-to-one teaching feedback is always provided, while in small groups, feedback is sometimes provided to the individual learners by the participants (SP, other learners, instructor).

One-to-One Encounter

In the one-to-one setting, the learner will enter a clinical exam room where an SP (and possibly a faculty observer) will be waiting. The learner will only interact with the SP until the end of the encounter. The SP will be prepared with a script pertaining to a specific medical problem. The learner will proceed with the medical encounter without prior prompting. If the SP is alone with the learner the encounter is almost always video recorded for potential review with a faculty member. At the conclusion of the medical encounter, the SP (and faculty observer if present) will provide feedback. The feedback should focus on one or two important points and include a balance of positive feedback and constructive critique. The learner should be given a second opportunity, if needed, to practice the skill incorporating the feedback received.

Feedback tips for all learners: begin the feedback by asking the learner what the experience was like for him/her. Typically, the learner will bring up at least some of the difficult issues that you wanted to discuss with him. Acknowledge any mistakes/omissions, weaknesses, but be sure to reinforce the positive elements of the performance as well. One 'lesson' is generally enough as learners cannot handle very much negative feedback. For very poor performances, it is generally better to simply acknowledge that the learner had difficulty and teach the 'skill' during the feedback time.

Additional tips for a struggling learner: if the learner responds to the opening question that he thought the interview went 'fine' when it did not, query him with something like: 'what was the best thing you did?' Then: 'how would you make it even better next time?' Acknowledge whatever they say and then add one appropriate additional suggestion of your own. Learners who have not yet developed adequate personal insight can benefit from this low key approach.

Small Group

The learner and the SP are at the front of the room before the small group. In this setting, the learner or the faculty facilitator may choose to intermittently interrupt the medical encounter role play, declaring a 'time-out' to prompt the audience for assistance as discussed in Technique 7. Generally a progressive interview model is used so that every learner gets a chance to participate in interviewing the patient. Alternatively, the facilitator may wait until the encounter is concluded to engage the entire group for comments, observations and feedback. In this situation, several oral simulations can be acted out in the same session.

Large Group

A faculty member may interview an SP to demonstrate an appropriate interview or other interpersonal interaction (noted in Technique 5). This could be followed by a discussion of how to elicit the patient's health beliefs, etc. during the clinical encounter. This activity could precede either the one-to-one or small group activities described above.

Time Required

Depends on the usage. Most one-to-one encounters last from a minimum of 10 minutes to a maximum of 30 minutes, mirroring the standard provider–patient interaction time. A group progressive interview generally takes about 30 minutes using the time-in/time-out technique.

Group Size and Structure

Depends on usage. For a demonstration, any size group is fine. For communication skill building, a small group of three to eight learners is optimal. For physical examination skill instruction, one-to-one teaching is preferable, accompanied by use of a video recording for later individual review.

Materials

Patient script; one or more trained performers; skilled facilitator; equipment if a physical examination is included.

Advantages

❑ SPs can closely imitate reality.
❑ Instruction can be concentrated on important aspects of the problem and eliminate irrelevant aspects.
❑ These learning strategies can be used when 'real' experiences are not readily available.
❑ SPs provide a standardized stimulus for learning or assessment.
❑ SPs can also act as evaluators and provide relevant feedback.
❑ This technique can also be use to help residents learn how to provide feedback, using standardized students, or to work in collaborative teams, using standardized health care providers.

Limitations

❑ Can be time consuming to develop cases and train actors or patients.
❑ Cost for paying actors or trained patients for performance.

At the end of an SP experience the impact can be extended with use of reflective writing or commitment to change.

Resources

Hall MJ, Adamo G, McCurry L, *et al.* Use of standardized patients to enhance a psychiatry clerkship. *Acad Med.* 2004; **79**: 28–31.

Makoul G. Commentary: communication skills: how simulation training supplements experiential and humanist learning. *Acad Med.* 2006 Mar; **81**(3): 271–4.

Morell VW, Sharp PC, Crandall SJ. Creating student awareness to improve cultural competence: creating the critical incident. *Med Teach.* 2002; **24**(5): 532–4.

Standardized Patient Case Development Protocol

1. **Directions**: select an actual case and include the relevant clinical, basic science, psychological, cultural, and/or ethical issues that are appropriate for the learners.
2. **Key words or phrases**: list no more than five or six words or phrases that describe the important learning points of the case.
3. **Case author(s)**: list the individual(s) involved with writing and/or revising this case, including the original author if case is revised.
4. **Case learning objectives**: describe in specific statements what the learners are to know or to be able to do when they have completed the case. When appropriate, specify level of learners.
5. **Presenting situation and instructions for learners**: provide a description of the learners' task and whatever clinical information the instructor wishes the learners to see prior to beginning to solve the case.
6. **Patient demographics**: state the age, sex, ethnicity, and socioeconomic status if relevant.
7. **Patient's personal presentation and emotional tone**: include details related to the patient's a) physical appearance (i.e. clothing, posture, facial expression, visual signs of illness); b) personal presentation (e.g. stylish, business-like, poor but neat, unkempt); c) interaction style (e.g. talkative, reticent, friendly); and d) emotional tone (e.g. depressed, confident, angry, worried, calm).
8. **Presenting problem (complaint, symptom, sign) and history of present illness**: describe current symptoms and immediate past history relevant to the presenting illness. Include pertinent information relating to a) chief complaint; b) symptoms in detail; c) history of present illness; d) any other medical conditions that may impinge upon the current complaint; and e) any 'problem behind the problem' (i.e. any emotional, psychosocial or cultural issue the patient is dealing with in addition to the presenting medical problem).
9. **Past medical history**: include a) relevant past medical history and family history; and b) information needed to answer 'all' medical questions likely to be asked by the learners.
10. **Psychosocial/personal/cultural history**: provide details in the areas of a) personal family history (e.g. abused as a child, grew up with mother only, both parents dead, etc.); b) educational background and occupational history; c) lifestyle (i.e. cultural background, living situation, significant others, etc.); d) patient risk factors (lifestyle risks such as use of alcohol, drugs, etc., relevant sexual history, any risk for suicide, environmental or other risk factors); and e) the data needed to directly answer questions related to any mnemonic being used (e.g. C-HEADDSS, ETHNIC, BATHE, LEARN, Q2).
11. **Physical examination**: portions of the physical examination that the learner is expected to perform (or gain information about) and any relevant findings.
12. **Laboratory data, x-rays, or other medical information**: describe this information, if applicable, and provide a description concerning how and where it will be incorporated into teaching or assessment activities.
13. **Treatment and long-term care**: specify the options for immediate treatment including referral or consultation, and how to prioritize care. When discussing drugs, classifications of drugs are generally better than specific drugs since specifics change rapidly. Rehabilitation, long-term care, home care, hospice, etc. should also be discussed as appropriate.
14. **Community resource issues**: if the case has objectives related to the need to engage community resources including public schools, welfare agencies, voluntary organizations (e.g. Cancer Society), specify.
15. **Prevention/health maintenance issues**: primary and secondary prevention issues and health maintenance issues related to the case should be listed and described.

TEACHING TECHNIQUE 9 Multi-Station Teaching Exercise

Description
The Multi-station Teaching Exercise (Teaching OSCE for short) is another creative way to efficiently and individually present a number of components of the cultural medicine curriculum to learners. It is very similar to the evaluation technique of the multiple-station examination. Learners move from station to station completing an activity at each station. Generally there are as many stations as learners, although it is acceptable to have one 'rest' station.

Uses
To help address multiple objectives in the cultural competence curriculum.

Process
1. Select stations to meet selected objectives (*see* table in Section 6 for example stations).
2. Prepare all materials for each session: computer stations, paper materials, video clips, standardized patients, station handouts, etc.
3. Plan the logistics for the session: obtain rooms; organize faculty, standardized patients, break snacks, etc.
4. As this is a teaching session, there must be feedback built into the experience.
   a) In-station feedback: if you can place a faculty member (or trained patient) at each station, then the feedback is built into the session. The tasks should be 15 minutes in length, with five minutes set aside for feedback.
   b) Group feedback: if you cannot place faculty at each station, then time to discuss the stations and insights can be scheduled within the multiple-hour session.
   c) Journal feedback: if all station activities are completed within the context of a journal, significant individual feedback can be provided following the session. However, time should still be scheduled for debriefing the multiple-station experience.

Time Required
Generally 15–20 minutes per station. Sessions lasting more than two hours should include a break (with refreshments) at the halfway point.

Group Size and Structure
A small group (five to eight learners) is optimal. With groups of 10–16 learners can rotate in pairs and still gain a significant amount of learning. With larger groups it is recommended to expend the resources on a multi-station evaluation exercise, particularly if resources are limited.

Materials
Exercises for each station; materials for each station; evaluation/feedback tools.

Advantages
Multi-station teaching exercises allow focused one-to-one teaching with multiple learners in a relatively short period. Instructors can focus each activity on a specific learning objective.

Limitations
Time and resources are the largest challenges, given the need for a multiple-hour block of time, and the availability of rooms (for example, if there are six learners, you will require two hours, six rooms, six exercises and several faculty members to sit at the stations and interact with the learners). A team is required to work together to develop and implement the Teaching OSCE.

Resources

Aeder L, Altshuler L, Kachur E, *et al*. The 'Culture OSCE': introducing a formative assessment into a postgraduate program. *Educ Health*. 2007 May; **20**(1): 11.

Altshuler L, Kachur E. A culture OSCE: teaching residents to bridge different worlds, *Acad Med*. 2001; **76**: 514.

Brazeau C, Boyd L, Crosson J. Changing an existing OSCE to a teaching tool: the making of a teaching OSCE. *Acad Med*. 2002 Sep; **77**(9): 932.

Green AR, Miller E, Krupat E, *et al*. Designing and implementing a cultural competence OSCE: lessons learned from interviews with medical students. *Ethn Dis*. 2007; **17**(2): 344–50.

Miller E, Green AR. Student reflections on learning cross-cultural skills through a 'cultural competence' OSCE. *Med Teach*. 2007 May; **29**(4): e76–84.

Rosen J, Spatz ES, Gaaserud AM, *et al*. New approach to developing cross-cultural communication skill. *Med Teach*. 2004 Mar; **26**(2): 126–32.

Catalysts

TEACHING TECHNIQUE 10 Progressive Disclosure Cases

Description

The progressive disclosure case is used to enhance participation and optimize educational impact without radical departure from a standard case-based session. Participants are asked to share impressions and knowledge as the case unfolds. At each discussion point in the case, the audience is asked to make decisions related to gathering data, diagnosis, treatment, education or follow-up. After each discussion, the actual data collected, diagnostic decision, care decision or education provided is shared. For each individual case, the goal is to focus on crucial aspects of the case and to strongly encourage active decision-making on the part of the audience.

Uses

To promote integration of cultural competence skills into problem solving and patient care; to illustrate additional data that should be collected when making a diagnosis and steps taken in negotiating a care plan.

Process

1. Planning:
    a) Select a topic that addresses an identified need for your learners.
    b) Determine the educational objective for the session. The objectives should relate to some important issue and guide the rest of the activities.
    c) Select an appropriate case: the case selected should be an actual one where you have all of the relevant information available (e.g. SP case development data).
    d) Select two or three discussion points from the case. At least one of these discussion points should relate to the selected focus for the session.
    e) Prepare a brief write-up to introduce the case, including all relevant information gathered prior to the first planned discussion point.
2. Opening the session: if not described in a prior session, the process of progressive disclosure should be presented.
3. Beginning the case: distribute the brief write-up prepared in advance. A verbal summary of this information is also provided at the beginning of the case.
4. Progressing through the case: as mentioned above, the case should have two to three discussion points. Below is a list of the steps that should take place during the conduct of an educational case with two discussion points.
    - Initial presentation of case leading into discussion point one.
    - Discussion point one: ask learners to write down their answer (1–2 minutes) or can use an audience response system and multiple-choice questions to gain the data (*see* Technique 11), and then conduct the discussion (4–5 minutes).
    - Summarize actual information gathered or actions taken at that point.
    - Additional information provided as a lead-in to discussion point two.
    - Discussion point two: summary of actual action taken at that point.
    - Review or debriefing of case focus.
5. Encouraging participation at the discussion points: the facilitator's role is to encourage interaction, so he/she should be careful not to dominate the discussion. The role is one of consolidating and clarifying what has been said. The facilitator's opinions should be

held until the end of the discussion. The facilitator should use the skills of facilitation and debriefing. At the end of each discussion, the facilitator should make a brief summary of suggested actions and may include his/her own suggestions at that time.

6. Session summary: the discussion leader should provide a one- or two-minute summary of the major learning points.

Time Required
Generally 20–30 minutes for a single progressive-disclosure case depending on the number of discussion points.

Group Size and Structure
Generally used in medium-sized or large groups.

Materials
The prepared case and electronic projection equipment.

Advantages
Encourages active participation and active problem solving.

Limitations
❑ Learning objective must be clearly outlined and case carefully selected.
❑ Participants must have adequate prior knowledge and/or experiences to tackle the case.
❑ There is no guarantee that all members will participate (process rules can help).

Note
Independent study prior to the session can ensure adequate knowledge prior to the experience. With large groups, use of an audience response system can help ensure a lively discussion, as disagreements are immediately evident as the responses are projected at the front of the room. Completion of a journal entry or commitment to change as part of the session or following the session can be used to expand impact.

Resource
Op't Holt TB. Problem-based and case-based learning in respiratory care education. *Respir Care Clin North Am.* 2005 Sep; **11**(3): 489–504.

TEACHING TECHNIQUE 11 Quizzes, Games, Polls, and Use of Audience Response Systems

Description

Quizzes, polls and audience response systems are all used for similar purposes – to focus learners' attention, or to help gage their level of knowledge or current awareness/attitudes on a given topic. Games are used to engage learners and promote active learning. Within the context of cultural competence training, a poll would be any method of assessing what the learners think or believe about the subject of interest, or it may examine their confidence or comfort caring for a designated group of persons or with a particular skill or task. A quiz is similar but its focus is generally on knowledge about a specific topic before or after a teaching/learning session. An audience response system (ARS) uses clickers to administer the polls or quizzes instantly. If you have an ARS available to you, use it. With most systems, the items are written into PowerPoint and when the system is initialized, the items shows on the screen. The learners then have 10 seconds to answer, with the seconds counting down on the screen in front of the room. When the countdown reaches zero, there is a brief pause and then the distribution of answers is displayed on the screen.

Uses

Quizzes: to assess knowledge of learners in relation to a specific topic of interest.
Games: to encourage learners to interact with the content and build enthusiasm for learning.
Polls: to gage awareness, attitudes, confidence in relation to a topic, culture, skills, etc.
ARS: to facilitate rapid administration of a quiz or poll and stimulate discussion among the learners on the topic of interest.

Process

1. Determine that a game, poll or quiz is the best method for stimulating interaction, focusing the learners, or reinforcing knowledge or attitudes discussed previously.
2. Develop the items, maximum of about 10.
3. Pilot test the items to ensure that they are clear, and that the correct answer (for any quiz) is definitive (agreed upon by experts).
4. Enter items into the ARS or make paper copies.
5. Use the game, poll or quiz within the session and make changes prior to the next usage, if required.

Time Required

Should be limited to no more than 10 minutes during a one-hour session.

Group Size and Structure

Any size group.

Materials

The game, poll or quiz (on paper or via ARS), the answers to any quiz or game questions.

Advantages

These methods provide a rapid way to assess learner need by gaining information about the current status of a group of learners in relation to knowledge or attitudes. If prepared in advance, these methods can allow tailoring of a session to the needs of the specific group; if administered using an ARS, they can stimulate discussion and allow for modifications within the session to meet learner needs.

Limitations

These methods are more useful for teaching knowledge and attitudes than for skill training. These techniques should be used sparingly to maintain their strength in gaining the interest and focus of learners on the session topic.

Resources

Eggert CH, West CP, Thomas KG. Impact of an audience response system. *Med Educ*. 2004 May; **38**(5): 576.

Glendon K, Ulrich D. Using games as a teaching strategy. *J Nurs Educ*. 2005 Jul; **44**(7): 338–9.

Johnson JT. Creating learner-centered classrooms: use of an audience response system in pediatric dentistry education. *J Dent Educ*. 2005 Mar; **69**(3): 378–81.

Latessa R, Mouw D. Use of an audience response system to augment interactive learning. *Fam Med*. 2005 Jan; **37**(1): 12–14.

Menon AS, Moffett S, Enriquez M, *et al*. Audience response made easy: using personal digital assistants as a classroom polling tool. *J Am Med Inform Assoc*. 2004 May–Jun; **11**(3): 217–20.

Miller RG, Ashar BH, Getz KJ. Evaluation of an audience response system for the continuing education of health professionals. *J Contin Educ Health Prof*. 2003; **23**(2): 109–15.

O'Leary S, Diepenhorst L, Churley-Strom R, *et al*. Educational games in an obstetrics and gynecology core curriculum. *Am J Obstet Gynecol*. 2005 Nov; **193**(5): 1848–51.

Schackow TE, Chavez M, Loya L, *et al*. Audience response system: effect on learning in family medicine residents. *Fam Med*. 2004 Jul–Aug; **36**(7): 496–504.

Streeter JL, Rybicki FJ. A novel standard-compliant audience response system for medical education. *Radiographics*. 2006 Jul–Aug; **26**(4): 1243–9.

TEACHING TECHNIQUE 12 Small Group Activities

Description

Small group activities are used to help students increase awareness, apply knowledge, and practice problem solving. Students are placed in small groups (5–10 learners) to complete a specified task. With medium-size groups (11–25) and large groups (over 25) of learners this method is used to supplement formal presentations by engaging the learners in active and critical thinking, typically around a case scenario. In general, the learners will exchange points of view concerning a topic or question and problem solve in order to arrive at a decision or conclusion. Most small group tasks are completed by groups of students without a faculty member to serve as facilitator. Typically one or more teachers rotate among groups to monitor progress.

Uses

To promote interactive learning (comprehension, analysis, synthesis) and skill acquisition related to multiple areas of competence including problem solving, professionalism, system-based practice, and interpersonal and communication skills.

Process

With this method, the small groups (5–10 learners) address a task designed by the instructor.
1. Prepare the task. The learning objectives and tasks must be clearly outlined. If a case is used, develop the questions or task in advance and provide it in writing to the group(s).
2. Divide students into small groups.
   a) If the learners will meet together many times, make permanent small groups. This facilitates development of collaborative skills. Caution: the lead instructor must 1. ensure that all groups know the process rules; 2. observe the groups for interaction issues; and 3. have intervention strategies for groups that struggle.
   b) If the learner group will meet only once, random groups are fine. Number off around the room to form the groups or, if the group is large (26+), develop a handout that pre-assigns learners to groups.
3. Provide task and process rules. Some standard process rules include:
   • everyone participates
   • all contributions are treated with respect
   • no one dominates the discussion
   • no side conversations
   • personal information revealed is kept within the room.
4. Completion of the activity (5–20 minutes).
   a) Instructor led: with this method, it can be helpful to start with think-write-share to give the learners a chance to talk to someone else before you start the general discussion. Caution: listen more than you speak, hold your comments until the end, facilitate learners talking to each other. Be careful that this process does not degenerate into multiple dialogues with instructor. *See* facilitation (Technique 16) for further hints.
   b) Facilitator led: trained facilitators do not need to be content experts – their job is to ensure that the group stays on task, finishes on time, and that all learners participate. When trained facilitators are used, this technique can be effective with very large groups of learners. *See* facilitation for further hints.
   c) Leaderless (without an assigned facilitator): with leaderless small groups, the instructor checks on each group periodically to ensure that each group understands the task and is addressing it appropriately. This variant is most effective when the total group has 25 or fewer participants (or multiple instructors) as it is challenging for one person to oversee more than three groups.
5. At the end of each small group activity or discussion, the whole group typically comes together for debriefing. Reflection and commitment to change can be used to expand impact.
6. Group discussion is often used within a larger session; one small group activity or discussion per hour of class is reasonable.

Time Required

Variable, depending on the assignment (generally 5–20 minutes for a single discussion).

Group Size and Structure

Small groups generally include 5–10 participants. With leaderless small groups (those without a trained facilitator) the technique is most effective when the total group has 25 or fewer participants. When trained facilitators are used with each small group this technique can be effective with very large groups of learners (requires many facilitators).

Materials

Stimulus materials (e.g. case study, web site activity, video clip, data to be reviewed, reading assignment, brief presentation or demonstration); clear description of small group task generally including discussion questions; trained small group facilitators or skilled large group leader.

Advantages

These techniques can promote exchange of ideas, recognition of mutual concerns, and encourage higher order thinking. Small group activities can foster teamwork and cooperation and can encourage active participation and active problem solving.

Limitations

Learning objectives and tasks must be clearly outlined or discussions can degenerate into conversations off the topic. Participants must have adequate prior knowledge and/or experiences to share in the group. Use independent study tasks to help ensure adequate pre-knowledge. Also, there is no guarantee that all members will participate in the discussion although process rules can help.

Resources

Haidet P, Morgan RO, O'Malley K, *et al.* A controlled trial of active versus passive learning strategies in a large group setting. *Adv Health Sci Educ.* 2004; **9**(1): 15–27.

Krueger PM, Neutens J, Bienstock J, *et al.* To the point: reviews in medical education teaching techniques. *Am J Obstet Gynecol.* 2004 Aug; **191**(2): 408–11.

Schweinfurth JM. Interactive instruction in otolaryngology resident education. *Otolaryngol Clin North Am.* 2007 Dec; **40**(6): 1203–14, vi.

Westberg J, Jason H. *Fostering Learning in Small Groups: A practical guide.* New York: Springer Publishing Company; 1996.

TEACHING TECHNIQUE 13 Think-Write-Share

Description

Think-write-share (or think-pair-share) is a rapid method to engage a medium-sized or large audience in thinking about a topic of interest, particularly sensitive or provocative topics. Learners are given a stimulus (interactive exercise, case, video clip, provocative quote, etc.) and asked to think for a minute or two, and then write down their thoughts either as bullet points or as complete sentences. This is typically followed by the opportunity to share with a partner (full participation) or to volunteer to share with the entire group (partial participation).

Uses

❏ To engage learners in thinking and talking about difficult topics (e.g. personal perception, unconscious bias).
❏ To help learners increase their personal awareness of the issues related to an area of concern (e.g. stereotyping, cross-cultural communication, health disparities).
❏ To accelerate learning and develop the habit of reflection and questioning of one's own assumptions.
❏ To provide a means for learners to process information on emotionally charged topics (e.g. gang violence, homelessness).

Process

1. Select the stimulus material for think-write-share based on the overall session objectives. As stated above, this may include an interactive exercise (e.g. eliciting opinions using an audience response system), case study (when the purpose is problem solving), video clip (e.g. of clinician–patient interaction), provocative quote, etc. In selecting video clips, short clips (less than five minutes) often generate better discussion than long pieces (like a movie or entire episode of a television program).
2. Provide directions for the activity. Tell the learners exactly how many minutes they will have to write and, if they are expected to share with someone, indicate how much time is provided for the sharing. Encourage the learners to share only as much of what they wrote as they feel comfortable sharing. Remind all students to hold in confidence anything shared in class.
3. With a medium-sized group, particularly an intact group, debriefing may follow directly after the writing portion. The facilitator needs to assess the level of trust within the group to ensure that most people will feel safe participating in the discussion.
4. With a large group, standard debriefing is used to bring the ideas together and provide take-home messages from the group's thinking.

Time Required

Generally five minutes or less is required for the thinking and writing portions of the activity. With the variant of think-pair-share, where learners share with a partner, add two to three minutes for the paired conversations prior to group debriefing. Debriefing generally takes 5–10 minutes.

Group Size and Structure

Any size group is fine. This is actually an ideal tool to enhance interaction with a large group (more than 50).

Materials

Computer and electronic transmission capability can be used to summarize points in the debriefing. For the exercise itself, the only requirement is paper and pencil for the participants.

Advantages

Learners, particularly within large groups, are difficult to engage and keep focused. When the topic is a 'soft' subject like interpersonal and communication skills, professionalism, advocacy or cultural competence, this problem is often exacerbated. The think-pair-share variant of this technique has been seen to take a large group of students who appear disengaged and transform them into an energized group of learners.

Limitations

Occasionally, students write very personal things during the 'write' portion that they may not feel ready to share, even with one other person. Others may be very superficial in what they write. Thus, learner readiness can be an issue. In any group of more than 100 there will probably be at least one who says the entire exercise is 'pointless' or 'a waste of time'. Occasionally, one of these students will attempt to disrupt the debriefing, so the more sensitive the subject matter, the more important it is to have a skilled facilitator.

Note

The writing portion can be expanded or deepened through use of written narrative and enhanced through use of commitment to change at the end of the session.

Resources

Network Learning Communities. http://www.eazhull.org.uk/nlc/think,_pair,_share.htm

Nolinske T, Millis B. Cooperative learning as an approach to pedagogy. *Am J Occup Ther*. 1999 Jan–Feb; **53**(1): 31–40.

Rao SP, DiCarlo SE. Peer instruction improves performance on quizzes. *Adv Physiol Educ*. 2000 Dec; **24**(1): 51–5.

Intensifiers

TEACHING TECHNIQUE 14 Commitment to Change

Description
At the end of a learning session, participants are asked to write down one or more changes they will make as a result of what they have learned during the session.

Uses
❏ To extend the impact of the session from the classroom into the work/clinical setting.
❏ To increase the chances that a positive change will be accomplished by participants.
❏ To study change and investigate facilitators and barriers to positive change in the work/clinical setting.

Process
Single Session Activity
As the participants move to complete the session evaluation form, call their attention to the 'commitment' item and explain the importance of making a commitment to positive change. To extend the impact you can also distribute index cards to record their commitment and take it home with them. If time permits, commitments can be shared among participants in groups with less than 20 people.

A small group variant in workshops (of two hours or more) would be to provide each participant with three cards upon which they would write their commitments to change. The cards would be collected, redistributed and read aloud by the group members. This helps to engage the whole group in a communal commitment to change. The leader may later type up all of the commitments and send the list to participants.

Longitudinal Intact Group (e.g. Residents, Semester Courses)
Commitments to change can be kept in a log or as part of a journal or portfolio. They can be reflected back upon by learners and discussed as part of an ongoing written reflection process. They can also be discussed as part of periodic meetings with instructors or advisors/mentors.

Follow-up Actions
With participants in a single session, follow-up is typically not feasible. Follow-up is often used with extended training programs (e.g. week-long intensive). Participants put their names on the commitment to change form and leaders can contact participants three to six months after the program to determine which of the planned actions have been taken and which have not. They discuss barriers and help the participants determine if the action is possible in their specific work/clinical setting. This data is also often used to assist in preparation of future training activities.

Time Required
About five minutes as part of the session wrap-up or the session evaluation.

Group Size and Structure
Any size group.

Materials

Evaluation forms with an item requesting a commitment to change. Index cards may also be used so participants can take their commitment with them. (*See* Section 6.)

Advantages

This is a quick way to extend the impact of a session into practice behaviors.

Limitations

It is very difficult to follow-up on the fulfillment of the commitments with a single session activity; it is important to follow-up when one of the session's objectives is to change practice behaviors of participants.

Note

With longitudinal intact groups, commitment to change can be combined with reflection or portfolios to track changes across time.

Resources

Dolcourt JL, Zuckerman G. Unanticipated learning outcomes associated with commitment to change in continuing medical education. *J Cont Educ Health Prof.* 2003; **23**(3): 173–81.

Lowe M, Rappolt S, Jaglal S, *et al.* The role of reflection in implementing learning from continuing education into practice. *J Cont Educ Health Prof.* 2007; **27**(3): 143–8.

Wakefield JG. Commitment to change: exploring its role in changing physician behavior through continuing education. *J Cont Educ Health Prof.* 2004; **24**(4): 197–204.

Wakefield J, Herbert CP, Maclure M, *et al.* Commitment to change statements can predict actual change in practice. *J Cont Educ Health Prof.* 2003; **23**(2): 81–93.

White MI, Grzybowski S, Broudo M. Commitment to change instrument enhances program planning, implementation, and evaluation. *J Cont Educ Health Prof.* 2004; **24**(3): 153–62.

TEACHING TECHNIQUE 15 Debriefing

Description

This technique is a type of guided large group discussion. It is frequently used after small group activities to ensure that the session objectives are met. This is the portion of most sessions where the facilitator ensures that the larger group is reflecting on the key objectives, and that they are achieving the desired awareness, knowledge, or skills. Depending on the objective of the session, this can be a time for the group (especially small groups) to honestly tackle difficult emotional or controversial issues. A superbly done debriefing can move individuals from initial to increased awareness, and toward a commitment to change.

Uses

- ❑ To deepen student learning related to an activity.
- ❑ To identify and discuss gaps in learner awareness/attitude, knowledge, or perceived skills as they relate to the activity.
- ❑ To ensure that learners get the take home messages (i.e. the central learner objectives).

Process

1. Pre-session preparation: the instructor must be very familiar with the small or large group task in order to be able to debrief effectively.
2. The instructor prepares prompts or questions in case they are needed. Some purchased activities have debriefing questions included in the kit that can be used or modified for the specific group of learners.
3. Rules for discussion need to be established for an inexperienced group. *See* hints below. Also, be sure to follow the guidelines provided for facilitation (Technique 16).
4. The debriefing: the leader's main role is to facilitate the debriefing process, rather than control it. When participants lack experience with debriefing, the facilitator may take on a stronger role to include:
   - ❑ use of an audience response system to capture opinions of all learners and structure discussion, especially if the group is very large;
   - ❑ facilitating discussion and highlighting conclusions;
   - ❑ summarizing outcomes and ensuring that learners receive the 'take-home' messages.

Time Required

Varies depending on topic and session objectives (typically 5–20 minutes.)

Group Size and Structure

Facilitator-led small groups enhance discussion, but debriefing can be done with any size group if the facilitator has appropriate knowledge and skill.

Materials

May use electronic means, whiteboard, or flip chart to record key discussion points.

Advantage

Debriefing is essential for learners to gain the maximum from any activity. This activity can be further extended with use of reflection or commitment to change

Limitation

The benefit of this activity is restricted only by the commitment of participants, the debriefing questions and the skill of the facilitator.

Resources

Owen H, Follows V. GREAT simulation debriefing. *Med Educ.* 2006 May; **40**(5): 488–9.
Stafford F. The significance of de-roling and debriefing in training medical students using simulation to train medical students. *Med Educ.* 2005 Nov; **39**(11): 1083–5.

TEACHING TECHNIQUE 16 Facilitation

Description
Facilitation is a key skill used in all sessions that include discussions or debriefing of activities. Effective and skilled facilitation is essential to teaching that goes beyond knowledge to application, skill building, and awareness/attitude enhancement.

Uses
❑ To enhance effectiveness of small and large group discussion; to assist learners to gain personal awareness in relation to any issue; to assist learners in effective interactions with each other so that they learn from each other.

Process
1. Prepare the session; objectives; pre-participation materials/activities; within session materials/activities. Make sure that materials/activities chosen will encourage discussion.
2. Prepare yourself intellectually (read and reflect prior to the session) and emotionally (remind yourself to listen and encourage; not react).
3. Establish an open atmosphere where learners feel comfortable sharing their ideas.
4. Establish and reinforce ground rules for discussion – sample rules might include:
    a) listen carefully to each other;
    b) be respectful of each other and the views expressed;
    c) as many people as possible participate – everyone gets to speak once if they choose to, before anyone speaks twice;
    d) no one monopolizes the discussion (not even the teacher);
    e) any private information that is revealed is NOT discussed outside the session.
5. In any session, the leader must attend to both the topic and the interactive process. Strategies include:
    a) ask open-ended questions, wait for learners to respond (don't answer your own questions);
    b) listen actively and non-judgmentally – maintain a neutral status as facilitator and help the group stay on track;
    c) prevent domination and interruption of discussion – ground rules are very useful here; with some controversial topics (such as racism in medicine), some conflict is an expected and important part of the learning process;
    d) model patience; ask for clarification and encourage learners to do it as well – if a comment is muddled you may need to paraphrase and ask them if you captured the meaning;
    e) ensure that differing views are heard and that no contributions are discounted – be prepared to engage a range of emotional responses (anger, sadness, resistance);
    f) note points of disagreement as well as agreement; accurately summarizing opposing views can be a very helpful discussion and learning tool;
    g) encourage learners to be aware of, and examine, their understandings, assumptions and values.

    Caution: listen more than you speak, hold your thoughts until the end, facilitate learner participation and interaction with each other; do not allow the discussion to degenerate into successive dialogues with instructor (or worse, an instructor monologue).
6. Some situations are particularly challenging. Below are ideas in relation to three of these.
    a) Difficult Learning Topics. Racism, sexism, health disparities, privilege, and power differentials are all highly volatile topics for discussion and exploration, yet they are essential components of learning in this curriculum. It is incumbent upon the facilitator that they be extremely comfortable with the material being discussed, that they have a strong capacity to work with group dynamics, and that they have fully immersed themselves in their own personal growth and self-challenges in these areas. Furthermore, the facilitator must be able to work non-defensively with learners in the face of anger,

sadness, resistance, and fear. The facilitator has a prime opportunity to model a constructive navigation of strong emotionally charged conversations.

b) Learner Resistance and Anger. The prepared facilitator scans all participants in the room, encouraging a wide range of participation. Learners will clearly be at different levels of knowledge, attitudes, awareness, and skills, and will differ in life experiences and encounters with oppression and disparity. Learner resistance may take the form of denying health disparities, for example, and be expressed in direct anger, sullen manipulation, or silent withdrawal. For those learners who seem particularly resistant or withdrawn, it is important to help them recognize where they stand in terms of these issues, to encourage self-reflection, but to carefully protect them from humiliation, from taking on too much before they are ready, and to the degree possible, from closing down. Other group members might be invited to share their experiences of resistance and/or anger as they face these issues, particularly if they are being asked to re-evaluate their own collusion with oppression or their own privilege in society.

c) Learner Sadness. The facilitator may be called upon to respond empathically to learners who are saddened and tearful from the material presented. An exploration of racial/ ethnic health disparities may awaken realizations and memories of how the learner's own family has been unduly impacted by morbidity, mortality and loss. Furthermore, sadness may arrive along with new understandings of the pervasive and pernicious nature and impact of racism and oppression. The facilitator can also engage the other participants to provide empathy, support, and understanding, as well as share their own emotional experience of learning activities.

7. If the group is very large and a difficult discussion is expected, a trained facilitator can be used. Trained facilitators do not need to be content experts – their job is to ensure that the group stays on task, finishes on time, and that all learners participate.

Time Required, and Group Size and Structure
Facilitation works with all groups, and time required varies.

Materials
A skilled facilitator.

Advantages
Use of facilitation skills and processes will add to the effectiveness of all sessions that encourage learners to interact with each other or with any other media (film, standardized patient, article, data report, etc.).

Limitations
An atmosphere of trust is required for discussions to be optimal learning experiences; for a sole teacher, facilitation of any session requires knowledge of the topic first and facilitation and other teaching skills second.

Resources
Azer SA. Challenges facing PBL tutors: 12 tips for successful group facilitation. *Med Teach*. 2005 Dec; **27**(8): 676–81.

Lekalakala-Mokgele E. Facilitation as a teaching strategy: experiences of facilitators. Curationis. 2006 Aug; **29**(3): 61–9.

Stafford F. The significance of de-roling and debriefing in training medical students using simulation to train medical students. *Med Educ*. 2005 Nov; **39**(11): 1083–5.

Steinert Y. Student perceptions of effective small group teaching. *Med Educ*. 2004 Mar; **38**(3): 286–93.

Westberg J, Jason H. *Fostering Learning in Small Groups: A practical guide*. New York: Springer Publishing Company; 1996.

TEACHING TECHNIQUE 17 Narrative and Reflective Writing

Description
Narrative writing is the use of creative writing to explore issues related to the competencies of professionalism, interpersonal and communication skills, and patient care. This technique begins with presentation of some form of dramatic stimulus material – short story, poem, video clip, movie, play, etc. The learners are then given a related writing assignment. Two types of assignments are common: 'point of view' in which students write their reaction to the stimulus materials from the point of view of one of the characters in the drama (generally patient, physician, other health professional, or family member); or a creative assignment to express their personal reaction to the stimulus in writing (sometimes these exercises allow other art forms – poetry, drawing, collage, clay sculpture). Reflective writing is similar but often focuses on personal reactions to and reflection on a real life event, and may include an analysis of their role in the event.

Uses
❏ To expand skills in listening, reflection, and written communication; to encourage learners to test their own assumptions and biases and increase awareness of these; to promote growth in understanding of self and others.

Process
1. Review session objectives to be certain that a narrative or reflective writing assignment can help meet the learner outcome objectives.
2. One key to an effective narrative writing assignment is compelling stimulus materials. Select the material carefully to help ensure that objectives will be met. Materials that can be viewed or read in a brief period of time (3–5 minutes) are generally preferred.
3. Develop the directions for the specific challenge or task for the students. For example: 'listen carefully to the following poem written from the point of view of a physician. After hearing the poem, you will have 10 minutes to write about your feelings in relation to the interaction, from the point of view of the patient.'
4. Plan how the learners will share their writing with each other – in pairs (using think-write-share) or in small groups.
5. Conduct the session. Be sure to remind students that it is not appropriate to discuss the writings of others outside the room without their express permission.
6. At the end of the paired or small group discussion the whole group typically comes together for debriefing. Commitment to change can be used to expand impact.

Time Required
Within a one-hour session, time varies (5–15 minutes) for writing (depending on the length of the required written product). Reserve time in the session (5–15 minutes) for learners to share their writings with each other in pairs and/or small groups. Longer assignments may be made as part of an independent study activity.

Group Size and Structure
Any size group is suitable for writing a brief narrative exercise. Exercises can be used as part of a journal or portfolio.

Materials
Paper and pencils; carefully selected stimulus materials.

Advantages
Narrative and reflective writing encourages learners to focus, listen carefully, and be able to examine a situation from multiple points of view. Positive change, particularly in awareness and attitudes, is based on reflection. The habit of reflection is essential to continued professional

growth throughout a career. Narrative and reflective writing are methods of requiring students to reflect and communicate their thinking.

Limitations

Some learners may be reluctant to share deep thoughts and may be very superficial in what they write. Feedback is helpful in encouraging learners to go deeper in their thinking and to be more creative in their expression.

Note

The long-term impact of single narrative assignments can be expanded if they are included as part of a portfolio.

Resources

Bartol GM, Richardson L. Using literature to create cultural competence. *J Nurs Scholarsh*, 1998; **20**(1): 75–9.

Bolton G. Narrative and poetry writing for professional development. *Aust Fam Physician*. 2007 Dec; **36**(12): 1055–6.

Bregman B, Irvine C. Subjectifying the patient: creative writing and the clinical encounter. *Fam Med*. 2004; **36**(6): 400–1.

Charon R. Narrative medicine: a model for empathy, reflection, profession and trust. *JAMA*. 2001; **286**: 1897–902.

DasGupta S, Meyer D, Calero-Breckheimer A, *et al*. Teaching cultural competency through narrative medicine: intersections of classroom and community. *Teach Learn Med*. 2006; **18**(1): 14–17.

Reilly JM, Ring J. Innovations in teaching: Turning point. *Fam Med*. 2003; 35(7): 474–5.

Winter RO, Birnberg BA. Teaching professionalism artfully. *Fam Med*. 2006 Mar; **38**(3): 169–71.

TEACHING TECHNIQUE 18 Student/Resident Presentation

Description

With this method the learner (resident or student) makes a formal presentation. It can be case-based, content-based, review of data or journal article, etc. The typical learner presentation blends presentation of an expanded case (expanded to address relevant issues in cultural competence) with a brief formal presentation.

Example assignment: 'the resident will prepare a case presentation of an encounter they found challenging in terms of some cultural and/or linguistic aspect of care. In the second half of their presentation, they will summarize research and/or theoretical sources that illuminate and expand upon the patient's health beliefs or healing traditions to the potential impact for the patient on his/her health, health care or access to care. Total presentation time is 12 minutes.'

Uses

❏ Increase self-reflection and self-awareness about cultural and linguistic challenges in the practitioner–patient relationship; increase learner confidence in discussing issues of cultural medicine with colleagues; promote knowledge of cultural medicine resources; increase understanding of the link between the behavior of health care providers and health disparities elimination.

Example Process

Instructor should modify the following process to fit exact objectives and assignment.
1. Learner selects a clinical case with significant cultural/linguistic issues, challenges, and/or successes, and makes use of resources provided by the instructor or selected by the learner to prepare the presentation.
2. The presentation will cover the following areas:
   * case description;
   * patient demographics;
   * any relevant health disparities data;
   * examples of significant verbal and non-verbal interchanges held with patient;
   * articulation of self-growth/self-awareness gleaned from the case;
   * summary of two or three relevant articles from cultural medicine literature that provide insight/guidance/support in navigating the cultural challenges in question.
3. Faculty and other residents/students provide feedback on the content and process.

Time Required

Approximately 10–15 minutes per learner (5 minutes for the case presentation and 10 minutes for the formal presentation).

Group Size and Structure

Works best with small groups. With larger groups, learners may work in pairs or in small groups, but the individual impact may be lower.

Materials

Presentation outline, visual aids, feedback form.

Advantages

Allows learners to explore health beliefs in depth; provides an opportunity to develop formal presentation skills; allows learner to develop a mini-expertise; learner presentations tend to engage other learners more effectively than faculty presentations – learners enjoy learning from each other and recognizing each other's knowledge and ability.

Limitations

With larger groups of residents or students it is challenging to find time in the curriculum for all learners to present. As with all techniques, this should be used sparingly and learners need individual feedback on their content and process. One-on-one meetings with an advisor or instructor to review presentations can be very valuable for students, time and resource permitting

Trackers

TEACHING TECHNIQUE 19 Journal

Description
A journal is a notebook in which experience is documented across time. Within the cultural competence curriculum, a journal can be a place to write the commitments to change at the end of each session. The key to the use of a journal is periodic review and reflection on growth across time. In the Cultural Competence Curriculum, Sessions 10, 20, and 30 are set aside for annual review of what each person has learned. If a journal is used with your group, this is the time for review of commitments and planning goals for future change.

Uses
To provide a place to record narrative and reflective writings, and commitments to change; to provide a means for learners to process emotionally charged events; to gain insight into and mentor learner growth through review of a journal kept across time and though periodic feedback provided to the learner.

Process
1. Determine the specific purpose and curricular objectives being met through use of a journal. Be sure that this is the right technique for your purpose and group.
2. Select a journal style and purchase them or simply create booklets tailored to your curriculum and learners.
3. Provide a standard format for the journal – an advantage of creating your own booklets. Following is the description of a journal used in a specific training program (called the Orientation Passport).
4. Distribute the journals and discuss the purpose of keeping their writings (reflections, narratives, and commitments to change, etc.) in a journal.
5. Periodically collect the journals, read them, and provide written and/or verbal input and feedback to each learner.

Time Required
The time required for a journal entry varies from five minutes to about 20 minutes, depending on the purpose of the entry and the length of the required written product.

Group Size and Structure
Journals can be used with any size group. However, it is extremely difficult for a single instructor to read more than about 10–12 journals, particularly if feedback to the learner is part of the process.

Materials
Computer and electronic transmission capability is recommended. Paper and pencil is okay.

Advantages
The journal is a convenient way of keeping commitments to change. Positive change, especially in awareness and attitudes, is based on reflection, particularly across time, and the journal, along with instructor feedback, encourages continued growth. If the writings collected in a journal focus on concrete plans for improvement or continued growth, it can increase the likelihood of positive change.

Limitations

Writing an entry in a journal takes time; thus, if use of a journal is adopted, classroom time must be set aside for preparing entries. Some learners may be reluctant to share deep thoughts and may be very superficial in what they write. Some learners think journals are stupid and may object to them as 'kid stuff'. You may want the group to decide how to record and keep track of their commitments to change: index cards collected at the end of each session; separate paper entries collected at the end of each session; or journals kept by the student and read periodically by an instructor.

Example Journal: Passport Documenting Learning During Orientation

The White Memorial Medical Center Family Medicine Residency Program in Los Angles is fortunate to have an entire month for intern orientation, of which many hours are dedicated to introducing and teaching basic elements of our culturally responsive health care curriculum. Offering a large portion of the cultural medicine curriculum from the start sends a message to the residents about the importance placed on this aspect of their training by the residency program. The Passport was developed as a tool for residents to record their orientation 'journey' and enhance their skills in self-reflection as they progress through the multiple learning activities. The Passport allows the learners to document their thoughts, impressions, and new learning, and eventually forms the foundation for their portfolio, which is developed over the three years of training.

Our Passport (*see* Section 6) includes thought-provoking quotations sprinkled among the pages. It also has a place on the back cover for signatures or 'passport stamps' as learners complete the various segments of the orientation curricular journey. It seems that the learners especially enjoy collecting these stamps along the way.

The learners are asked to answer specific reflection questions at the completion of each cultural medicine curriculum activity. The journals are collected at the completion of each week for faculty members to read and provide comments on the individual reflections. This serves as an opportunity to engage in a feedback loop with the learners regarding the struggles and challenges they write about. It also keeps them on task, and provides faculty an opportunity to assess the degree and depth to which the learners are engaging with the material offered.

As described in the portfolio technique of this curriculum (Technique 20), we hope that this Passport will serve as a document that learners can turn back to in the future to remind them of important lessons they want to hold on to over the course of their professional lives, as well as to serve as a milestone from which they have grown and developed over the course of their training and beyond.

Our Passport changes each year along with our schedule and shifting of teaching activities. You are encouraged to use our Passport as a model you can tailor to your program's unique curriculum and schedule.

Resources

Blake TK. Journaling: an active learning technique. *Int J Nurs Educ Scholarsh*. 2005; **2**(1): article 7.

Plack MM, Driscoll M, Blissett S, *et al*. A method for assessing reflective journal writing. *Journal of Allied Health*. 2005; **34**(4): 199–208.

Shapiro J, Kasman D, Shafer A. Words and wards: a model of reflective writing and its uses in medical education. *J Med Humanit*. 2006; **27**(4): 231–44.

TEACHING TECHNIQUE 20 Portfolio

Description

A learner portfolio is a factual description of and reflection on the learner's accomplishments. Portfolios contain documents and materials including annual individual learning plans, projects, presentations, written reflections, and letters from patients, which collectively suggest the scope and quality of performance. It can empower the learner to reflect on areas like communication, teamwork, and professionalism, and to work toward enhancement of these areas. A portfolio can also document improvement efforts.

In the context of building cultural competence, the learner portfolio may simply be a longitudinal collection of individual reflections or commitments to change, or it may include other documents. It may be organized around the specific objectives of a Cultural Competence Curriculum or use the Accreditation Council for Graduate Medical Education (ACGME) competencies or other national/specialty/school-wide set of goals, or it may combine the two.

Assessment of learner portfolios can be used as part of either formative or summative evaluation. Portfolios can be useful in gaining information on mastery of competencies that develop across time. At the student level these competencies might include such things as documentation of various patient encounters, culturally competent case write-ups, and use of scientific evidence in patient care. At the resident level these competencies might include such things as reflections on patient encounters or other experiences, and descriptions of activities including: practice-based learning and improvement activities, teaching activities, patient advocacy, hospital committee service, and progress in the resident's research/scholarly project.

Uses

❏ To document growth in relation to specific objectives or areas of competence.
❏ To enhance personal professional development through periodic review of past reflections.
❏ To provide information for mentor/advisor meetings to supplement standard evaluations like end-of-rotation ratings and periodic examinations.

Process

1. Develop the objectives for the portfolio – be very clear how the portfolio will be used to reinforce and assess learning.
2. Develop clear requirements for the portfolio, which must minimally include a) table of contents and b) descriptions of each item that might include a reflective statement about why that particular entry was selected and what it demonstrates (*see* example list of entries below).
3. Establish deadlines for entries and space them throughout the program.
4. In programs longer than one week, instructors should review the portfolios periodically, providing guidance and encouragement to the learners. This review is extremely important in encouraging continuing professional growth, acknowledging accomplishments and stimulating new plans (e.g. semi-annual review of resident portfolios and development of new learning plans.

Time Required

Variable depending on the portfolio requirements.

Group Size and Structure

Portfolios can be used with any size group. However, it is extremely difficult for a single person to read more than about 10–12 portfolios, particularly since feedback to the learner is part of the process.

Materials

Computer and electronic transmission capability is recommended for the e-portfolio. Notebooks, dividers, paper, etc. are required for the paper portfolio.

Advantage

Provides a means to gather extensive data on competencies that need to be reviewed across time, like cultural competence, professionalism, and practice-based learning and improvement.

Limitation

Portfolios are time consuming to create and to review. The portfolio as a series of reflections as described in the 'reflection' section is very feasible, and almost identical to a journal. For the more traditional portfolio, less is more; that is, do not be too ambitious in terms of the number of items to be included – better to have the learners focus on a small number of carefully selected items that are mindfully and thoughtfully completed.

Example Cultural Competence Entries that Address ACGME Competencies

❏ Knowledge: scores from any locally prepared test of knowledge related to the cultural competence curriculum; learner plan for enhancement/improvement; documentation of completion of plan.

❏ Patient care: reflection of an unexpected positive connection with a patient from a differing background; or a challenge overcome with a 'challenging' patient.

❏ Interpersonal and communication skills: review of a video for culturally responsive communication and discussion of how will use in own care; review of video of self interviewing a patient; narrative related to a story, poem, visual image, movie, etc.

❏ Professionalism: reflections on self-awareness exercises like those on the PBS Race Website; annual letter to self discussing growth in past year and goals for achieving excellence next year.

❏ Practice-based learning and improvement: reflection of unexpected negative feelings/ stereotypes and a plan to enhance future encounters; commitments to change with discussion of annual review.

❏ System-based practice: reflection on the diversity of their patient panel (groups included and missing); description of a policy study; reflection on a specific medical error and the changes in the system that need to be made to avoid this type of error in the future.

Resources

Carraccio C, Englander R. Evaluating competence using a portfolio: a literature review and web-based application to the ACGME competencies. *Teach Learn Med*. 2004; **16**(4): 381–7.

Challis M. AMEE Medical Education Guide No. 11: portfolio-based learning and assessment in medical education. *Med Teach*.1999; **21**: 370–86.

Chisholm CD, Croskerry P. A case study in medical error: the use of the portfolio entry. *Acad Emerg Med*. 2004 Apr; **11**(4): 388–92.

Clay AS, Petrusa E, Harker M, *et al*. Development of a web-based, specialty specific portfolio. *Med Teach*. 2007 May; **29**(4): 311–6.

Gordon J. Assessing students' personal and professional development using portfolios and interviews. *Med Educ*. 2003; **37**(4): 335–40.

Lawson M, Nestel D, Jolly B. An e-portfolio in health professional education. *Med Educ*. 2004 May; **38**(5): 569–70.

McMullan M, Endacott R, Gray MA, *et al*. Portfolios and assessment of competence: a review of the literature. *J Adv Nurs*. 2003; **41**(3): 283–94.

Parbooshingh J. Learning portfolios: potential to assist health professionals with self-directed learning. *J Cont Educ*. 1996; **16**: 75–81.

Tiwari A, Tang C. From process to outcome: the effect of portfolio assessment on student learning. *Nurse Educ Today*. 2003; **23**(4): 269–77.

TEACHING TECHNIQUE 21 Reflection and Self-Assessment

Description

A written exercise where learners are asked to examine their performance over a specific time period, identifying strengths, potential areas for growth and specific plans for making improvements. These exercises may also include completion of self-assessment rating forms. Completion of the written exercise must be accompanied by a one-to-one meeting with a faculty member for maximum benefit.

Uses

❑ To encourage the habit of self-reflection and self-critique vital to life-long learning and professional excellence; to help learners extract the maximum from learning experiences; to accelerate learning; to gain diagnostic information about learners' approaches to reflection and self-assessment, the content of the self-assessments, and plans for future improvement.

Process

This is a one-to-one process with the following steps:

1. Discuss the purpose of reflection (*see* uses above) and the reasons to record reflection in writing (we quickly lose ideas that are not recorded; recording our thoughts allows us to track them across time).
2. Provide a standard format for reflections tailored to your session/course/rotation objectives. Below are some sample items that might be included in a reflection:

Sample Set 1

End of unit on cultural context of health care for medical students. Summarize the main learning points for you personally, during this unit:

❑ Summarize how you have grown in relation to the school's learner outcome objectives during this unit.
❑ Describe at least one area requiring continued growth in relation to objectives of this unit.
❑ Outline a specific plan for how you will continue to progress in the area identified.

Sample Set 2

Reflection for a resident or medical student in a clinical rotation.

❑ Over the next week, take a few minutes each day to reflect upon your performance in this rotation. Keep brief notes of your thoughts, e.g. what in your performance went really well, what could have gone better, what might you do differently next time?
❑ At the end of the week, sit down and complete the items below.
❑ Make an appointment to meet with instructor to discuss your reflection and self-assessment.
Items for reflection:
❑ briefly describe three things that you have done really well during this experience;
❑ briefly describe up to three things that you still need to work on;
❑ make a list and after each item write a one-sentence plan for how you might work on that item.

3. Collect your own notes on any observed performance of the learner.
4. Meet with the learner to discuss the content of their reflection as well as the process of reflection and critique. Note the level of thinking (complexity and depth) in the reflection and the quality and specificity of the plan. Help the learner clarify his/her thinking and planning. Stay as positive as possible. You want to praise progress and try to redirect the learner in areas in which he/she is struggling.

Time Required

Meeting time will vary from five minutes to several hours (typically 15–20 minutes) depending on the purpose of the self-assessment and the length of the required written product.

Group Size and Structure

Any size group for completing self-assessment rating forms. For written reflection and self-assessment exercises, it is extremely difficult for a single instructor to meet with more than 10–12 learners to provide the one-to-one feedback that is part of the process for periodic reflection and self-assessment.

Materials

Computer and electronic transmission capability recommended. Paper and pencil okay.

Advantages

Positive change, particularly in awareness and attitudes, is based on reflection. The habit of reflection and self-assessment is essential to continued professional growth throughout a career. Discussion of relative strengths and weaknesses encourages recognition of past changes and openness to continued growth. Reflection, added to the skill in developing concrete plans for improvement for continued growth, increases the likelihood of positive changes.

Limitations

Instructor must model change based on reflection and self-assessment and should share this with learners. Learner readiness can be a challenge. Learners must be open to the process of true reflection, realistic self-assessment, and the potential need to change. Trust between instructor/advisor/mentor and the learner is required for this process to be optimal. Many learners (and instructors) need guidance in developing this skill.

Note

Reflection and self-assessment can be enhanced through review of video-taped samples of performance or through expansion of the reflection process accomplished by use of ongoing commitment to change forms and a portfolio.

Resources

Chambers N. Close encounters: the use of critical reflective analysis as an evaluation tool in teaching and learning. *J Adv Nurs.* 1999; **29**(4): 950–7.

Davis DA, Mazmanian PE, Fordis M, *et al.* Accuracy of physician self-assessment compared with observed measures of competence: a systematic review. *JAMA.* 2006 Sep 6; **296**(9): 1094–102.

Gianakos D. Self-reflection, learning, and sharing mistakes. *Pharos Alpha Omega Alpha Honor Med Soc.* 1999; **62**(4): 33–4.

Hodges B, Regehr G, Martin D. Difficulties in recognizing one's own incompetence: novice physicians who are unskilled and unaware of it. *Acad Med.* 2001; **76**(Suppl.): S87–9.

Latham CL, Fahey LJ. Novice to expert advanced practice nurse role transition: guided student self-reflection. *J Nurs Educ.* 2006 Jan; **45**(1): 46–8.

Murray-Garcia JL, Harrell S, Garcia JA, *et al.* Self-reflection in multicultural training: be careful what you ask for. *Acad Med.* 2005 Jul; **80**(7): 694–701.

Regehr G, Hodges B, Tiberius R, *et al.* Measuring self assessment skills: an innovative relative ranking model. *Acad Med.* 1996; **71**(10 Suppl.): S52–4.

Riley-Doucet C, Wilson S. A three-step method of self-reflection using reflective journal writing. *J Adv Nurs.* 1997; **25**(5): 964–8.

Section 5

Cultural Exercises

Cultural Exercises:
Overview and Table of Contents

Overview

In this section you will find the description of a sampling of exercises used to help build cultural competence. Most are short exercises (15 minutes or less), but one is a nine-hour online curriculum. Many of these learning activities are recommended as a primary or alternative exercise for use in one of the 33 sessions in the curriculum.

Table of Contents

Below is a listing of the exercises with a notation of the Cultural Competence Curriculum (CCC) objectives that relate to the exercise, the session number (if any) in which it is used, and the page number where it is found within this section.

EXERCISE 1 Autobiography

Description

This activity is an important part of team building. Learners prepare an autobiography and turn it in. Students should be given several days to complete the assignment. Prior to this session, the leaders of the cultural competence curriculum should read all of the student biographies and prepare their own to share. Following is a sample assignment.

Instructions for students: we want you to write an autobiography (4–6 pages) that shares your perspectives on your personal development, cultural context, and family history. We want you to tell us your story. This is NOT a personal statement like the one submitted for medical school or residency, NOR is it a resumé of accomplishments. We want to hear about the people, events and experiences that shaped your life. It will have four parts: 1. family background and cultural context (1–2 pages); 2. significant events/experiences that shaped who you are (1–2 pages); 3. family strengths, health issues and risk factors (1 page); and 4. how you ended up in medical school and within your chosen specialty (1 page). Learners are encouraged to include the motivations behind their becoming a health professional.

In class, learners share elements of the autobiography with each other as part of team building.

Use

To begin to build awareness and knowledge in relation to culture, healing traditions, and health beliefs and to help learners become familiar with each other and grow together as a learning community.

Activity Objectives

Upon completion of this exercise, the learner will be better able to:
1. discuss his/her cultural heritage, gender, class, ethnic-racial identity, sexual orientation, disability, age, and spirituality; to reflect on it and describe it (Objective 2 – awareness)
2. identify healing traditions and beliefs, including ethno-medical beliefs of own family and those of peers (Objective 8 – attitude, skills)
3. exhibit comfort when conversing with colleagues about cultural issues (Objective 9 – attitude).

Time Required

Preparation of the autobiography is estimated to take each learner several hours. Preparation time for instructors is about 20 minutes per autobiography. Encouraging comments should be written on each, particularly noting any insights in cultural areas. Sharing can be done in small groups, but at least an hour should be scheduled for sharing and discussion.

Group Size and Structure

A small or medium-sized group (5–25 learners) is optimal; if the group is larger it should be divided into small groups for the activity and discussion.

Materials

Autobiography assignment, faculty autobiography to share with group.

Advantages

Has the potential of bringing a new group close together very rapidly through the power of sharing each other's stories.

Limitations

As with all independent assignments, learners must take the task seriously, they must also be open to listening to each other with respect.

Methodology

1. Provide learners with the autobiography assignment and explain that everything we do

emanates from who we are (our personal wiring and our stories). Stories help us understand ourselves, and others. As part of building a community we will each write our story and share it with others in the group.

2. Have learners submit their autobiographies in a timely manner, so that the lead faculty can read all of them prior to the session.

3. This exercise is typically used as part of orientation when team building is most crucial. Judgment forms quickly in terms of perceptions as to the nature and worthiness of any group experience. A good start sets the stage for everything that follows. The leaders of the Cultural Competence Curriculum set the tone. Being approachable, warm, setting learners at ease and communicating excitement for the curriculum, and your role in it, is a good beginning. You want the learners to look forward to working together within the Cultural Competence Curriculum.

4. Share your story first (be brief); then divide the learners into small groups to share with each other. If the group is small (5–8 learners) try to schedule enough time so that everyone has a chance to share with the whole group. If the group is larger, typically you will need several groups.

5. In the small groups each person should have a minimum of five minutes to talk. Some groups choose to make copies and share their written autobiographies with each other. That should be the choice of the group. The group should be reminded to share with each other information regarding their families' health practices and beliefs.

EXERCISE 2 Chicken Soup

Description
This exercise invites learners to recall specific home remedies used within their families and to explore the importance of culturally congruent care. It was first shared with us by Marya Cota, PhD.

Use
To promote understanding of one's own and others' healing traditions and health beliefs.

Activity Objectives
Upon completion of this exercise, learners will be better able to:
1. describe their own cultural heritage in relation to healing traditions and health beliefs (Objective 2 – awareness, skill)
2. describe historical models of common health beliefs among the families of their colleagues (Objective 7 – knowledge)
3. identify and appreciate healing traditions and beliefs of patients and/or their families, including ethno-medical beliefs (Objective 8 – awareness)
4. elicit additional information about ethno-medical conditions and ethno-medical healers (Objective 8 – Skill).

Time Required
Approximately 15 minutes.

Group Size and Structure
Small or medium-sized group is ideal (5–25 learners), if group is larger it can be broken into smaller groups, each with a facilitator.

Materials
Flip chart and tape, marker for each learner.

Advantages
Uses personal stories to help learners deepen their understanding of their own cultural heritage; helps learners appreciate the traditions of their colleagues.

Limitations
The knowledge portion is limited by the experiences of those in the room; there may not be a breadth of traditions represented.

Methodology
1. Preparation: a number of pieces of flip chart paper are taped to the walls in the classroom prior to the start of the session.
2. Task: each participant is given a marker and asked to think back to when they were very young. When someone was sick in their household, what were the family remedies used to help the sick family members to feel better? As they recall these, they are to note them on one of the large sheets of paper on the walls.
3. Debriefing: the facilitator reads some of the family remedies aloud, inviting the participants to more fully explain their remedy. It can be interesting to ask them whether they felt the remedy was effective, and whether they would still use it today. The discussion should be upbeat, lively, full of curiosity and respectful humor. Participants may want to share the degree to which the healing tradition is 'typical' for their own ethnic background.
4. Conclusion: at the conclusion of the exercise, ask the participants why they think this exercise was selected for today's learning session, and what they take with them as a learning point for the cultural medicine curriculum. Hopefully, they will suggest that it reminds them of the comfort of family remedies, the wisdom of the elders, how much of medical treatment happens outside of the doctor's office, and that a 'culturally congruent' cure is often very important to people, especially when they are ill.

EXERCISE 3 Drawing Differences

Description

Learners are asked to recall a time in their life when they felt different from others and capture that difference in a crayon drawing. The drawing is done in silence. This exercise was first shared with us by Shelly Harrell, PhD.

Use

To introduce difference, bias and stereotyping; to help learners recognize their own potential for bias and stereotyping.

Activity Objectives

Upon completion of this exercise, learners will be better able to:

1. discuss the dynamics of difference and appreciate the emotional impact of being treated as 'different'
2. identify the risks and benefits of stereotyping
3. value the importance of curiosity, empathy, and respect in patient care and the importance of continuous growth as a healer (Objective 12 – attitude)
4. recognize their own potential for bias and stereotyping, be able to identify their own stereotypes and biases and explore how their attitudes, biases and stereotypes affect clinical encounters, clinical decision-making and quality of care (Objective 13 – awareness, knowledge).

Time Required

Approximately 25–30 minutes (5 minutes for instructions and distribution of materials; 5–10 minutes for individual drawing activity; 10–15 minutes for debriefing).

Group Size and Structure

Small or medium-sized group (5–25 learners); if group is larger it can be broken into smaller groups, each with a facilitator.

Materials

Table space for each learner to draw, crayons (or other drawing supplies) and paper, flip chart or similar equipment for debriefing.

Advantages

Uses a different media, drawing, to creatively increase learner awareness.

Limitations

Being asked to draw is not a typical assignment for a health sciences student or resident and might be met with resistance. Emphasize that artistic quality is not the issue here, rather the drawing is a vehicle to capturing a particular life scenario from a certain period in the past.

Methodology

1. Each learner is provided with a piece of paper and crayons. They are invited to close their eyes and the facilitator recites the following instructions:

   'Think about a time in your life when you felt different in some way. It may be the first time that you felt different from others. As best you can, picture the situation including where you were, who you were with, and feelings associated with the experience of difference.'

2. Learners are given a minute or two in silence to conjure the memory. Next they are instructed to capture that memory of difference in a crayon drawing. The drawing is done in silence and typically takes about five minutes.
3. To open the discussion with a small group, the facilitator might begin the debriefing by sharing his/her experience of difference. With a large group, the facilitation might start

with asking learners to share their drawing and the feelings they had with the person next to them. This keeps the audience active in the discussion (a variant of think-write-share).

4. The facilitator then invites volunteers to share their experiences with the entire group, their drawings, and the feelings associated with those experiences. The facilitator collects these experiences in a two-column table displayed to the group. The table should have the following headings: 'Differences' and 'Feelings'. Continue listing until everyone who wants to share has done so, or until about 10 or 12 examples are collected.

5. Next, the group as a whole is invited to make observations about the lists. A common observation is that the feelings associated with differences are predominately negative. The group is asked to consider and discuss why this might be the case, even though the facilitator was careful not to request a recollection of the first 'negative' experience with difference. This should lead the facilitator into a discussion of the dynamics of difference and stereotyping. Some suggested debriefing questions are listed below.

6. The final discussion should relate to the impacts of stereotyping on patient care.

Some Discussion Questions

1. What are your observations? What feelings are not in the table and why?
2. What are some other experiences that we may have heard from others?
3. What is it about childhood differences that really stand out? (The need to fit in, to be part of the group, human need to belong, the things that are most powerful are things you cannot change, makes you vulnerable.)
4. What is the emotional impact of being treated differently over and over (e.g. being a member of an oppressed group)?
5. Describe/discuss the primary benefit of stereotyping (e.g. that categorizing people and ideas is a natural cognitive adaptation to living in a complex world).
6. List three risks to the patient who has been stereotyped by the provider.
7. What can providers do to keep a stereotype from becoming unrecognized prejudice and unintentional discrimination?
8. Based on the insights you gained in this exercise, describe one thing that you are going to do differently in your interactions with patients.

Resource

van Ryn M. Research on the provider contribution to the race/ethnicity disparities in medical care. *Med Care*. 2002; **40**(1 Suppl.): I140–51.

EXERCISE 4 Genogram Exercise

Description

Learners complete and present a personal genogram (a diagrammatic family history that extends the concept of a family tree to include relationships, health risks, and protective factors). A genogram is essentially a pictorial or symbolic representation of a family history. More specifically, the genogram activity offers the learner an opportunity to explore and share their own family history including any relevant family issues such as cultural and religious/spiritual background, immigration, quality of relationships, loss, and milestones. Learners are encouraged to include family strengths, health issues, and risk factors, and the motivations behind their becoming a health professional. Learners are invited to include photographs and family artifacts to illustrate their presentation.

Use

❏ To gain a depth of understanding about own family and cultural history and that of classmates, including health risks and protective factors.
❏ To promote team development through depth of knowledge and understanding of each member.

Objectives

Upon completion of this exercise, the learner will be better able to:
1. discuss his/her cultural heritage, gender, class, ethnic-racial identity, sexual orientation, disability, age, and spirituality; to reflect on it and describe it (Objective 2 – awareness)
2. identify healing traditions and beliefs, including ethno-medical beliefs of own family and those of peers (Objective 8 – attitude, skills)
3. exhibit comfort when conversing with patients/colleagues about cultural issues (Objective 9 – attitude).

Activity Objectives for all Variations

Upon completion of this exercise, participants will be able to:
1. complete a genogram for patient's family as part of health history taking
2. recognize and describe the impact of family health history on their own development and viewpoints on health and health care
3. discuss multiple cultural practices and health beliefs within families.

Additional Activity Objective for Small Group Variation

Increase awareness of similarities and differences among learners to facilitate development of a peer support system.

Time Required

About two hours required for genogram preparation and approximately 45–60 minutes for each genogram presentation and discussion.

Group Size and Structure

The genogram activity can be implemented in:
❏ a small group of learners (2–8) in which everyone takes turns to present their family history to the rest of the group
❏ a large group of learners (9 or more) in which learners pair up and share their genogram with one other student
❏ one-on-one learning in which learner shares his/her genogram with a faculty member.

Materials

Genogram instruction sheet, transparencies, overhead projector and/or LCD projector are required for large or small group settings (box of tissues recommended for oral presentations).

Advantages

This exercise has the potential of bringing a new group close together very rapidly through the power of extended sharing. When conducted in a small group or paired learner setting, participants tend to bond closely as the assignment demands taking risks and sharing personal information with others. This technique also helps build psychosocial history-taking skills.

Limitations

Very time consuming, not all programs have 45–60 minutes for each learner to share his/her genogram with the group; this can be an extremely intense and very emotional exercise and thus requires a skilled facilitator, particularly in the small group variant.

Methodology

The instructor and other group leaders must set confidentiality parameters clearly when initially describing the exercise. In small residency training programs, the faculty might want to inform learners that the presentations are not confidential, and that learners are invited to be as open as possible, but encouraged to share only that information that they feel comfortable about being shared with faculty members outside the session. This allows instructors to transmit important information garnered about learners from the genogram presentations to the faculty as a whole, helping to illuminate learner's backgrounds. With groups larger than nine, perhaps a more appropriate guideline would be 'what is shared here, stays here', emphasizing confidentiality of genogram material.

When the genogram assignment is made, a faculty member may want to model a presentation (20–30 minutes) for the group. This can be done if the group is meeting multiple times, and there is sufficient time in the schedule to allow for an extended introduction of the assignment.

Exercise Variations
Exercise 1

(No in-class time)
Learners complete a genogram and submit it to the instructor who can provide written feedback. The learner may present the genogram orally, one-on-one to an instructor, or simply submit the genogram with a written narrative describing the salient aspects.

Exercise 1 + Sharing in Pairs

(1–2 hours in-class time)
Using a think-pair-share model, learners present their genograms to one other learner from the large group setting. The pairs of learners might be encouraged to find a quiet, more private location where they can talk. This exercise can then be followed by a large group discussion or debriefing of what was learned in the exercise.

Exercise 1 + Small Group Sharing

(45–60 minutes per person in-class time)
Each of the participants, along with the faculty coordinating the workshop, presents their genograms to the rest of the group. Genograms can be photocopied on overhead transparencies or prepared on posters or LCD projected slides. Group participants are invited to ask questions, make observations and comment on the genogram presentations. As learners are presenting their genograms, emphasis should be placed on eliciting information regarding culturally relevant health practices and beliefs.

An additional option is to invite learners to conclude their presentations with a view of their own personal vulnerabilities to and strategies for coping with stress, as well as a description of what faculty and colleagues can do to support them in stressful times. The instructor is invited to ask questions, make observations, and comment on the genogram presentation.

Exercise and Reflection

Self-reflection underlies an effective cultural medicine curriculum. Therefore, consider a written reflection component at the conclusion of the genogram exercise, independent of the variation implemented. This can be part of an ongoing journal. Learners might be invited to respond to the following prompts:

❑ For individuals: what was it like to prepare and present (if relevant) your genogram? Any surprises in terms of the information you collected (self, family, or cultural background) or your reactions? What do you see as your own health risk and protective factors? What is the most important thing you learned from this exercise?

❑ Additional questions for small groups: what was it like to listen to colleagues' presentations? What did you learn from them?

Cautionary Notes

❑ Upon receiving the assignment, some learners react with alarm to what feels 'invasive'. It can be explained that this helps create empathy for the experience of their patients during a history and physical exam.

❑ Some learners will assume this is a benign 'no-brainer' assignment, and are later surprised at the intense emotions the preparation and sharing/presentation can precipitate.

❑ As with many awareness exercises, there will be a range of emotional responses from participants, ranging from great emotional expression to relative detachment. The facilitator should be prepared to discuss these responses in the group or individually at a later time as necessary.

❑ Small group: in the small group variation, this is a time-consuming and emotional exercise that requires a skilled facilitator to successfully manage the intensity. The number of presentations should be limited to a maximum of three in each half-day session.

Extending the Experience

Completing a genogram for a patient is an effective means for understanding the impact of a patient's family history and social context (great activity for first and second year medical students). In a modified form, it can be used in a rotation that focuses on areas like adolescent medicine, geriatrics, behavioral medicine, and addiction medicine.

Take-Home Messages

Culture clearly impacts family dynamics, health beliefs, and practices. Understanding one's own family history and dynamics is an essential component of becoming a compassionate, culturally responsive practitioner. Understanding your colleagues' cultural and family background can help build positive and empathic teams.

Resources

Northwestern University. *Understanding Genograms*. Available from: Sociology Central. *Genograms*. http://www.sociology.org.uk/as4fm3a.pdf

This website was originally created to assist students in the Family Communication class at Northwestern University. It explains the 'multigenerational transmission of communication patterns'. It also contains explanations of symbols used to identify individuals and their relationships to each other.

Zamudio A, Hill K. Building closeness, understanding, and tolerance among residents: the family genogram. *Fam Med.* 2004; **36**(2): 625–6.

EXERCISE 5 Imagery Exercise

Description
Learners participate in a guided imagery exercise that is followed by debriefing and discussion of stereotypes.

Uses
❏ Help learners to recognize their own potential for bias and stereotyping (Objective12 – awareness).
❏ Help learners identify and appreciate how clinician bias and stereotyping can affect interactions with patients, families, communities, and other members of the health care team (Objective 13 – awareness).

Objectives
Upon completion of this exercise, participants will be able to:
1. describe how limited information produces stereotypical thinking
2. acknowledge the learner's own tendencies to stereotype
3. acknowledge specific stereotypes held by them toward particular groups.

Time Required
Approximately 10 minutes to conduct the imagery exercise and approximately 15 minutes to debrief the exercise.

Group Size and Structure
Small group, large group, one-to-one.

Materials
List of descriptors for facilitator.

Advantage
Can be used with very large groups to help raise awareness in relation to unconscious stereotypes and biases.

Limitations
Requires a very skilled facilitator to gain maximum effect; learner readiness can be a problem; need to be prepared for resistant learners.

Process
Exercise (10 minutes)
Instruct participants that they will be doing an 'imagery exercise' so as not to taint the process by telling them that it is a stereotype exercise. Ask the learners to clear their minds and close their eyes and imagine the individuals who will be described for them. They are encouraged to conjure up the most detailed and textured images of each individual as they can, including physical characteristics, dress, setting, and context. They are informed that the facilitator will provide additional descriptive information about each individual, and they should let their mental image develop in their mind's eye. The descriptors are then read slowly, with approximately 30 seconds pause between each one. When completing one image and moving to the next, the facilitator asks the participant(s) to gently erase the image from their mind and prepare to imagine the next one. At the conclusion, the facilitator asks participants to open their eyes and describe their experience (*see* debriefing questions below).

Descriptors
The descriptor clusters are as follows, although facilitators could certainly develop their own to supplement or replace these (*see* below for teaching points):
African-American Woman
❏ single mother

❏ extremely wealthy
❏ Chief of Cardiology at (name a prominent hospital)

Teenage Girl
❏ born in El Salvador
❏ lives in New York City
❏ attends a high school for performing arts

Gay Man
❏ Japanese ancestry
❏ father of two
❏ just celebrated his 82nd birthday

Female Lawyer
❏ American Indian
❏ Chippewa Nation
❏ 64 years old
❏ works for a multinational corporation

White Male
❏ world-class athlete
❏ requires a wheelchair for mobility

Chinese American Man
❏ addicted to drugs
❏ second year family medicine resident (this descriptor can be altered to mirror your audience)

Teaching Points for Descriptor Sets

The descriptors included in the Imagery Exercise were designed to specifically challenge participants' pre-existing assumptions or stereotypes by including a heavy dose of the unexpected. They were elaborated step by step to elicit stereotypes in a wide array of categories, hopefully illuminating both the automatic nature of stereotyping, as well as the breadth of categories of individuals about which we harbor preconceptions.

1. The African-American Woman descriptors challenge assumptions about gender, race, professional roles and socioeconomic status.
2. The Teenage Girl descriptors draw out stereotypes about immigrant status and about adolescents. These descriptors take less dramatic turns than the previous descriptors, allowing participants a more 'gentle spin' on these stereotypes.
3. The Gay Man descriptors are often the most challenging for participants. These descriptors were designed to challenge assumptions about sexual orientation, ethnicity, and family role, and to address ageism.
4. The Female Lawyer descriptors also challenge assumptions about age, ethnicity, gender and employment. The 'Chippewa Nation' descriptor was added specifically because, for most participants, it is unfamiliar to them and adds little to their ongoing elaboration of the image. This provides an opportunity for a discussion about what we do with information about others for which we have either little understanding or context.
5. The White Male descriptors challenge assumptions about ethnicity and gender for majority group members, as well as assumptions about physical abilities.
6. For the Chinese American Male descriptors, the instructions suggest tweaking the final descriptor to mirror the audience who is partaking in the exercise. This brings the exercise closer to home, challenging one's attitudes and assumptions about 'the other' versus individuals similar to oneself professionally. This descriptor also explores biases about drug abusers.

Debriefing (15 Minutes)

The debriefing for this exercise is similar for one-on-one, small, or large group learning. With small or large group learning, think-pair-share methodology is helpful in allowing everyone in the room the opportunity to share their experience of the exercise with someone else, and to hear another learner's experience as well.

The objective of the debriefing period is to allow the learners to reflect on their experience of the exercise, and to learn more about the process of stereotyping in a personal way. Examples of debriefing questions are as follows.

❑ What was your experience of this exercise?
❑ What references did you use to come up with your mental images? (Common references include family, friends, colleagues, acquaintances, and media images.)
❑ What were your initial images and how were they similar/different from peers' images?
❑ Were there certain descriptor clusters that were more challenging for you? Why?
❑ What did you learn about yourself from this exercise?
❑ What stereotypes might patients have of you?
❑ How might practitioner bias and stereotyping affect interactions with patients, families, communities, and other members of the health care team?

The discussion after the exercise should focus on the universality of stereotyping as a cognitive strategy to order a complex world. Learners should be encouraged to keep a mindful eye on the assumptions they are making of others. It is also helpful to remind them that stereotyping works both ways in the doctor–patient relationship, such as when patients see a female physician enter the room and assume it is their nurse. This can engender a broader discussion of stereotyping in the doctor–patient relationship and its role in contributing to health disparities; and stereotyping and its affect on communication among the health care team.

Take-Home Messages
❑ Stereotyping is unavoidable. Stereotyping is a normal human process for organizing massive amounts of information we take in every day.
❑ Patient care decisions made based on our stereotyping contribute to health disparities and decrease the quality of care.
❑ Stereotyping tends to happen more frequently and rigidly when one is under stress (such as time pressure), and when one has limited information.
❑ It takes conscious effort to manage our stereotypes.

Cautionary Note
Learners should not 'beat themselves up' for having relied on stereotypes, but should consider when stereotyping can become problematic and learn strategies to manage their stereotypes.

Resources
Dovidio JF, Gaertner SL, Kawakami K, *et al.* Why can't we just get along? Interpersonal biases and interracial distrust. *Cultur Divers Ethnic Minor Psychol.* 2002; **8**(2): 88–102.
Pinderhughes E. *Understanding Ethnicity, Race and Power.* New York: The Free Press; 1989.

EXERCISE 6 Implicit Association Test (IAT)

Description

Learners individually take the IAT, which is designed to discover unconscious or automatic biases. There are several tests to choose from, including tests on various ethnic groups, race, gender, religion, and skin tone. Instructor carefully selects one or two IATs, depending on the specific objectives of the session or the curriculum. The learners can then, either individually or as a small group, discuss any increase in their awareness, or why they may not have found any differences in their responses.

Uses

❏ Help learners to recognize their own potential for bias and stereotyping (Objective 12 – awareness).
❏ Help learners identify and appreciate how clinician bias and stereotyping can affect interactions with patients, families, communities, and other members of the health care team (Objective 13 – awareness).

Activity Objectives

Upon completion of this exercise, learners will:
1. be able to state any automatic thoughts they may not have shared with others
2. name their implicit biases (of which they may previously have been unaware) (Objective 12 – awareness).
3. describe differences between bias, stereotypes, prejudice, and discrimination (Objective 1 knowledge).

Time Required

Approximately 10 minutes to complete each IAT and 10 minutes to debrief the exercise.

Group Size and Structure

Since this is an independent study exercise it can be used with any size group. The process is different depending on group size (small group, large group, one-to-one).

Materials

Learners will need a computer with a high-speed internet connection. Handouts of the relevant topics from the Tolerance.org website should also be made readily available.

Advantage

Can be used with very large groups to help raise awareness in relation to unconscious stereotypes and biases.

Limitations

Requires a very skilled facilitator to gain maximum effect; learner readiness can be a problem; need to be prepared for resistant learners.

Process

1. Become thoroughly familiar with the Project Implicit website. The IAT Background and FAQ sections are particularly useful. Select one or two IATs based on your objectives. Personally take each of the IATs that you plan to assign. Absorb your results and be ready to share them with your students.
2. Have learners go to the IAT demonstration site and complete the assigned exercises (each takes about 10 minutes). https://implicit.harvard.edu/implicit/demo/
3. On the Project Implicit website the researcher quotes Dostoyevsky. Using this quote could be a powerful way to open a session that uses the IATs. You may want to read it twice, once using man and once using woman:

'Many years ago, Fyodor Dostoyevsky wrote:

> Every man has reminiscences which he would not tell to everyone but only his friends. He has other matters in his mind, which he would not reveal even to his friends, but only to himself, and that in secret. But there are other things which a man is afraid to tell even to himself, and every decent man has a number of such things stored away in his mind.'

Modified (woman):

> 'Every woman has reminiscences which she would not tell to everyone but only her friends. She has other matters in her mind, which she would not reveal even to her friends, but only to herself, and that in secret. But there are other things which a woman is afraid to tell even to herself, and every decent woman has a number of such things stored away in her mind.'

> 'These lines from Dostoyevsky capture two concepts that the IAT helps us examine. First, we might not always be willing to share our private attitudes with others. Second, we may not be aware of some of our own attitudes. Results on the IAT may include both components of control and awareness.'

https://implicit.harvard.edu/implicit/demo/background/posttestinfo.html

4. Debriefing: the willingness of learners to examine their own possible biases is one of the most important steps in changing the way discrimination increases health disparities in our society. This exercise can sometimes bring up confusion, anger, and/or sadness for the learner when they discover biases they may have thought they never had. The instructor should be prepared to process these emotions and help the learner focus on what they can do to prevent these biases from negatively affecting their behaviors. The tutorial on the website can be reviewed after the learner completes the test. This can be found at: http://www.tolerance.org/hidden_bias/tutorials/index.html

Resources

Dovidio JF, Gaertner SL, Kawakami K, *et al*. Why can't we just get along? Interpersonal biases and interracial distrust. *Cultur Divers Ethnic Minor Psychol*. 2002; **8**(2): 88–102.

Gladwell M. *Blink: The power of thinking without thinking*. New York: Little Brown and Company; 2005.

Nosek BA, Banaji MR, Greenwald AG. *Project Implicit*. Available from: http://implicit.harvard.edu/; 2006.

Tolerance.org website: http://www.tolerance.org/hidden_bias/index.html Discusses stereotypes, prejudice and discrimination and links to the various IATs.

EXERCISE 7 Neighborhood Study

Description

This exercise encourages the learner to spend time in the community in which their patients live. It encourages learners to examine the community factors that contribute to variability in population health and to develop a map of a portion of the area. Community characteristics to look for:

❑ Economic: where do people work, shop, are there signs of unemployment or decay (e.g. empty stores, boarded up buildings, vacant lots, abandoned vehicles, homeless people); signs of prosperity (types of cars, clothing, shops, services, etc.)?
❑ Education: primary/secondary schools, libraries, colleges, proprietary schools
❑ Food: liquor stores versus grocery stores, family-owned restaurants versus chains versus fast food
❑ Health care and medical: hospitals, health-related businesses, alternative providers
❑ Housing: types, condition of buildings and yards
❑ Interactive: where do people 'hang out'
❑ People: ethnic groups, ages, gender mix
❑ Political: county or city courthouse, government buildings
❑ Recreational: what recreational facilities are available, and who participates
❑ Religious and expressive: churches/synagogues/mosques/other places of worship
❑ Topographic and geographic major features, obstacles and physical barriers (e.g. freeways, hills)
❑ Transportation: condition of roads, public transportation
❑ Violence: signs of gang activity or crime (e.g. trash, graffiti, people with evidence of past injury)
❑ Pollution: environmental health risk factors.

Uses

❑ To promote learner familiarity with the community and all elements listed above.
❑ To examine factors in the community that might affect health and health care disparities.
❑ To encourage learner value of the importance of social determinants and community factors on health.

Activity Objectives

Upon completion of this exercise learners will be better able to:
1. value the importance of diversity in health care and address the challenges and opportunities it poses (Objective 3 – attitudes)
2. value the importance of social determinants (e.g. education, culture, socioeconomic status, housing and employment) and community factors on health, and strive to address them (Objective 6 – attitudes).

Time Required

Approximately one hour for the neighborhood study, one-half hour for each small group to make a map, collage of photos or other activity to describe experience, and one-half hour for in-class discussion.

Group Size and Structure

Small or medium-sized group (5–25 learners); if group is larger it should be divided into small groups for the activity and discussion.

Materials

Map of community, assignment of sections of the neighborhood for each pair (or trio) of learners, art supplies.

Advantages

Interactive task that requires learners to experience the community with their five senses (sight, hearing, touch, smell, and maybe taste).

Limitations

As with all independent assignments, learners must take the task seriously.

Process

1. Map out a section of the community surrounding the medical center and assign each pair/trio of students a segment that includes several residential and several non-residential blocks.
2. Provide instructions: 'With your partner(s), tour the assigned community area and note the community characteristics listed. Your community survey will be enhanced if you are able to speak with members of the community (e.g. school teacher, local pharmacist, store owner, priest, local clinic personnel, or people living in the community), shop at a store, or eat at a restaurant.'
3. Ask learners to prepare a product and be prepared to discuss their findings and product at the next meeting. The product depends on the specific objective of the session. It can be a community map, photo collage, poem, essay, etc.
4. Debrief the group. The debriefing should be based on your specific program objectives related to the community context of health and health care.

Note

This exercise can be extended through use of narrative or reflective writing and journal or portfolio.

Resources

Eugenia E, Blanchard L. Action-oriented community diagnosis: a health education tool. *Int Q Commun Health Educ.* 1991; **11**(2): 93–110.

Sloane P, Slatt L, Ebell M, *et al.* (editors). *Essentials of Family Medicine.* Baltimore: Lippincott Williams & Wilkins; 2002.

Neighborhood Study: Instructions for Learners

Directions

With your partner(s), tour (for approximately 1 hour) the assigned community area, exploring in particular those features listed below. Your community survey will be enhanced if you are able to speak with members of the community (e.g. school teacher, local pharmacist, store owner, priest, local clinic personnel, or people living in the community), shop at a store or eat at a restaurant.

Community characteristics to look for include:

- ❏ Economic: where do people work, shop, are there signs of unemployment or decay (e.g. empty stores, boarded up buildings, vacant lots, abandoned vehicles, homeless people); signs of prosperity (types of cars, clothing, shops, services, etc.)?
- ❏ Education: primary/secondary schools, libraries, colleges, proprietary schools
- ❏ Food: liquor stores versus grocery stores, family-owned restaurants versus chains versus fast food
- ❏ Health care and medical: hospitals, health-related businesses, alternative providers
- ❏ Housing: types, condition of buildings and yards
- ❏ Interactive: where do people 'hang out'
- ❏ People: ethnic groups, ages, gender mix
- ❏ Political: county or city courthouse, government buildings
- ❏ Recreational: what recreational facilities are available, and who participates
- ❏ Religious and expressive: churches/synagogues/mosques/other places of worship
- ❏ Topographic and geographic major features, obstacles and physical barriers (e.g. freeways, hills)
- ❏ Transportation: condition of roads, public transportation
- ❏ Violence: signs of gang activity or crime (e.g. trash, graffiti, people with evidence of past injury)
- ❏ Pollution: environmental health risk factors.

At the completion of your Neighborhood Study, prepare a group product, typically a Community Map (this should take approximately 30 minutes). Be creative, have fun. Your product should express your understanding of the community. Be as creative as you wish in drafting important features of your Community Map. Since this is a creative project, your product does not have to be a Community Map. It could be a photo collage, a series of sketches, a narrative, a poem, an essay, etc. Art supplies are available for your use. Be prepared to discuss your findings and your Community Map at our next meeting.

Activity Objectives

Upon completion of this exercise, learners will be better able to:

1. value the diversity in our community, and discuss the challenges and opportunities it poses to health and health care in our community;
2. value the importance of community factors and social determinants (e.g. education, culture, socioeconomic status, housing, and employment) on health and strive to address the challenges in our community.

EXERCISE 8 Sorting People (Matching Faces with Races)

Description
Learners group pictures of people into 'racial categories' based strictly on physical appearance. The exercise is completed on the PBS Race website: http://www.pbs.org/race/002_SortingPeople/002_00-home.htm

Uses
❏ Define, in contemporary terms, race and ethnicity (Objective 1 – knowledge).
❏ Become aware of own ethnic-racial identity, be able to reflect on it and describe it (Objective 2 – awareness, skill).
❏ Value the importance of curiosity, empathy, and respect in patient care (Objective 11 – attitude).

Activity Objectives
Upon completion of this exercise, learners will be able to:
1. identify the physical traits they use to classify race and understand that racial classification is a highly subjective process
2. discuss our evolving understanding of race
3. acknowledge the importance and confusion of self-identification
4. describe the importance of curiosity, empathy, and respect in patient care.

Time Required
Approximately 20 minutes (5 minutes for the exercise, 10 minutes to answer the questions, 5 minutes to review the 10 facts about race).

Group Size and Structure
Any size group.

Materials
Computer with internet access; handouts of some of the key points of the exercise.

Advantages
Exercise can be completed prior to class; inherent interest in the exercise; increases readiness of learners to discuss issues of bias and stereotyping.

Limitations
Requires learner readiness to question their own prior assumptions and examine how we define race and culture.

Process
This exercise can be done individually or as a group. Learners will sit in front of a computer and follow these instructions:
1. Go to the following website: http://www.pbs.org/race/002_SortingPeople/002_00-home.htm
2. Select the 'Sorting People' link, and complete the exercise.
3. Answer questions in 'Human Diversity'.
4. Read 'Where Race Lives'.
5. Click on each of the Ten Facts about race to learn more.

Debriefing: learners might complete a written reflection at the completion of the exercise. In class, learners will debrief with the instructor, or as large group.

Evaluation can be done both through learners' level of participation in the debriefing process, as well as through the administration of a paper or online quiz in relation to the PBS: Ten Facts of Race found on the website at: http://www.pbs.org/race/.

Instructor Note

The instructor should be well prepared to engage learners in a discussion of the cross-cultural issues involved. They must become very familiar with the website and video cases and be able to guide the discussion to the pertinent issues. For a more detailed explanation for instructors, please see discussion guide at the PBS website: http://www.pbs.org/race/images/race-guide-lores.pdf

Resources

Adams M, Blumenfeld WJ, Castaneda R, *et al. Readings for Diversity and Social Justice: An Anthology on Racism, Sexism, Anti-semitism, Heterosexism, Classism and Ableism.* New York: Routledge; 2000.

Pinderhughes E. *Understanding Ethnicity, Race and Power.* New York: The Free Press; 1989.

Race – The Power of an Illusion. Available from: http://www.pbs.org/race/

EXERCISE 9 'Think Cultural Health' Online Learning Program

Description
There is an e-learning website developed by the US Department of Health and Human Services, Office of Minority Health. The program is entitled 'A Physician's Practical Guide to Culturally Competent Care' and can be located at www.thinkculturalhealth.org. This nine-hour training program is divided into three overall themes: 1. Culturally Competent Care, 2. Language Access Services and 3. Organizational Supports. It provides a thorough overview of the CLAS Standards. Furthermore, the training elements are built around clinical and organizational cases that highlight cultural and linguistic clinical and organizational dilemmas and challenges. The program is creative and engaging, with brief videos of the introductory cases. It offers interactive opportunities for reflecting on the material presented, as well as numerous links for further reading and exploration of themes of interest. Each theme has three one-hour modules.

Theme 1 – Culturally Competent Care
1. Overview of Culturally Competent Care discusses the rationale for and benefits of cultural competency, and introduces the Culturally and Linguistically Appropriate Services (CLAS) standards.
2. Cultural Competency Development includes a definition of cultural competency, explains fact-centered and attitude/skill-centered approaches, and describes frameworks for developing cultural competency.
3. Patient-Centered Care and Effective Communication present models for effective physician–patient communication.

Theme 2 – Language Access Services (LAS)
1. Importance of LAS.
2. Models to provide LAS (interpretation and translation).
3. 'Working Effectively with an Interpreter' introduces the triadic interview process and provides guidance for working effectively with interpreters.

Theme 3 – Organizational Supports
1. Importance of environment/climate.
2. Assessing your community.
3. Building community partnerships.

Uses
To supplement and enrich the Cultural Competence Curriculum that a local program is able to provide. With a small staff, and few class hours available, this makes efficient use of classroom time.

Activity Objectives
This nine-hour Continuing Medical Education (CME) program has many objectives compatible with the Cultural Competence Curriculum in relation to awareness, attitudes, and knowledge, and helps prepare learners for skill development sessions. It addresses issues with each of the following objectives: 1, 9, 10, 13, 14, 21, 22, 23, 24, 25, 27, 28.

Time Required
Nine hours of computer-based training, three hours of in-class discussion.

Group Size and Structure
Any size group.

Materials

Computer with internet access; handouts of some of the key points of the exercise.

Advantages

Twenty-first century students are very comfortable with online exercises; exercises can be completed any time during the week at the convenience of the learner; makes efficient use of class time. There is no cost for this activity.

Limitations

The online curriculum may not match the specific objectives of the local Cultural Competence Curriculum. Nine hours may be a lot to ask of busy learners.

Process

1. Instructors must complete the nine-hour curriculum and be ready to discuss key points. You may want to print out pages with key concepts that you wish to discuss in class.
2. Assign learners one theme (3 modules) per week. They need to go to the website at www. thinkculturalhealth.org, register, and then they can return to the site at any time.
3. Weekly debriefing: a weekly group discussion time provides the forum for talking together as a group about the web-learning experience and the specific content in the 'theme of the week'. These meetings can serve not only as helpful debriefing sessions, but help to keep learners accountable for finishing each theme in a timely manner.

Resource

Office of Minority Health, US Department of Health and Human Services. *Cultural Competency Curriculum Modules (CCCM)*. Available from: http://www.thinkculturalhealth.org/

Section 6

Evaluation Tools

Evaluation Tools:
Overview and Table of Contents

Overview

In this section you will find copies of tools currently in use in relation to the curriculum. It is our intent that this section will grow in both volume and sophistication of tools over time. The current tools are listed below.

Table of Contents

Cultural Medicine Questionnaire

Instructions: please fill out this questionnaire to the best of your ability.

Date: _____

Specialty: _____

Level (Year of Training): _____

Circle the best answer.
1. Which the following terms is the LEAST important to include in your definition of the term 'culture'.
   a) language
   b) sexual orientation
   c) health beliefs
   d) race
   e) stereotype
2. How relevant are your attitudes, beliefs, and stereotypes to patient care?

1	2	3	4	5
not at all	a little	moderately	quite relevant	very relevant

3. How important is it to work to eliminate health care disparities?

1	2	3	4	5
not at all	a little	moderately	quite important	very important

For each of the items below, check how often you have performed each of the activities within patient care. Use the following key to select the best option.

Key:	Never		Monthly		Daily
	1	2	3	4	5

Q.	Items	Never		Monthly		Daily
		1	2	3	4	5
4.	Recognized a personal bias when caring for a patient.					
5.	Integrated complementary and alternative therapies into treatment plans.					
6.	Worked with a live interpreter.					
7.	Used remote telephonic interpretation.					
8.	Witnessed the effect of bias and stereotyping on clinical encounters and clinical decision-making.					
9.	Elicited a cultural, social, and medical history, including a patient's health beliefs and model of their illness.					
10.	Used negotiating skills in shared decision-making with a patient.					
11.	Witnessed that bias and stereotyping within my profession can affect interactions within the health care team and impact the quality of care provided.					
12.	Asked patients what their beliefs are about their illness and what they think might help.					
13.	Discussed cultural issues with a patient or colleague.					
14.	Asked patients about their use of complementary and alternative therapies.					
15.	Included patients' beliefs and traditions when developing patient care plans.					
16.	Worked to reduce your biases and those of others to lessen the effects of bias on clinical care.					

For each of the items below, check how often you have performed each of the activities within your studies. Use the following key to select the best option.

Key:	Never		Monthly		Daily
	1	2	3	4	5

Q.	Items	Never		Monthly		Daily
		1	**2**	**3**	**4**	**5**
17.	Examined/discussed national data on health, health care disparities and/or quality of care.					
18.	Examined/discussed local data on health, health care disparities and/or quality of care.					
19.	Discussed the underlying causes of health care disparities and the barriers to eliminating them.					
20.	Worked with a community agency that serves to enhance health care and eliminate disparities.					

For each of the following statements, state your level of agreement by placing a check in the column using the following key:
SD = strongly disagree; D = disagree; SLD = slightly disagree; SLA = slightly agree; A = agree; SA = strongly agree.

Q.	ITEMS	SD	D	SLD	SLA	A	SA
21.	Infant mortality is higher for Hispanics than for African-Americans.						
22.	Health care disparities can result, at least in part, from clinician bias.						
23.	I have reflected on my own cultural context (gender, age, disability, class, ethnic-racial identity, spirituality, sexual orientation) as it relates to my role as a clinician.						
24.	I am committed to addressing the challenges and opportunities posed by diversity in health care.						
25.	The patient's race/ethnicity, culture, and class can impact clinical decision-making.						
26.	I am able to describe how access, historical, political, environmental, and institutional factors (including racism and discrimination) impact health and underlie health and health care disparities.						
27.	I can discuss the social determinants of health including the impact of education, culture, socioeconomic status, housing, and employment.						
28.	I am interested in working to address the social determinants and community factors affecting heath and health care disparities.						
29.	I can describe the health practices and beliefs that are common in the community my program serves.						
30.	There is an inherent power imbalance between the physician and patient that affects the clinical encounter.						
31.	I have the skills required to conduct a community study including examination of population health criteria, social mores, cultural beliefs, and health needs.						

32. The CLAS Standards are directed toward which group?
   a. Patients
   b. Physicians and other providers
   c. Community-based organizations
   d. Health care organizations
33. When interviewing a patient with the assistance of an interpreter, it is best to speak directly to the interpreter and then turn your attention to the patient in anticipation of the patient's response.
   a. True
   b. False
34. Give the definition for any one of the following culturally responsive interviewing and patient care mnemonics: LEARN, ETHNIC, C-HEADDSS, or Q2.

Cultural Competence Curriculum Objectives Versus Test Item Numbers from the Cultural Medicine Questionnaire

No.	Objective	Test Items
1.	Define, in contemporary terms, race, ethnicity, and culture, and their implications in health care.	1
2.	Become aware of own cultural context (heritage, gender, class, ethnic-racial identity, sexual orientation, disability, age, spirituality), be able to reflect on it and describe it.	23
3.	Value the importance of diversity in health care and address the challenges and opportunities it poses.	24
4.	Identify patterns of national data on health, health care disparities, and quality of health care, and be able to discuss.	17, 21
5.	Discuss the epidemiology of health and health care disparities for the local community using *Healthy People 2010* and other resources.	18, 24
6.	Value the importance of social determinants and community factors on health and strive to address them.	27, 28
7.	Describe historical models of common health beliefs (for example, illness in the context of 'hot and cold'), and identify questions about health practices and beliefs that might be important in a specific local community.	29
8.	Identify healing traditions and beliefs of patients and/or their families, including ethno-medical beliefs. Ask questions in a non-judgmental manner to elicit patient preferences; listen and respond appropriately to patient feedback about key cross-cultural issues. Elicit additional information about ethno-medical conditions and ethno-medical healers.	12, 14
9.	Discuss race, ethnicity, and culture in the context of the medical interview and health care. Exhibit comfort when conversing with patients/colleagues about cultural issues.	13, 18
10.	Recognize and describe institutional cultural issues and discuss for own institution. Discuss CLAS Standards.	32
11.	Value the importance of curiosity, empathy, and respect in patient care and the importance of continuous growth as a healer.	13
12.	Recognize their own potential for bias and unavoidable stereotyping, identify their own stereotypes and biases and explore how their attitudes, biases and stereotypes affect clinical encounters, clinical decision-making and quality of care.	2, 4, 8
13.	Identify and appreciate how clinician bias and stereotyping can affect interactions with patients, families, communities, and other members of the health care team, and the link between effective communication and quality care.	11
14.	Describe the impact of the patient's context (cultural heritage, gender, class, ethnic-racial identity, sexual orientation, disability, age, and spirituality) on clinical decision-making.	25
15.	Describe strategies for reducing physician's own biases, and those of others, and demonstrate strategies to assess, manage, and reduce bias and its effects in the clinical encounter and in clinical practice.	16
16.	Describe the inherent power imbalance between physician and patient and how it affects the clinical encounter.	30
17.	Recognize and describe how access, historical, political, environmental, and institutional factors (including racism and discrimination) impact health and underlie health and health care disparities.	19, 26
18.	Identify how race, ethnicity, and social determinants of health (e.g. education, culture, socioeconomic status, housing, and employment) affect health and health care quality, cost, and outcomes.	–
19.	Identify and discuss the contributors to disparities (patient, provider, health care system, and society) and discuss the challenges and barriers to eliminating health disparities.	–
20.	Describe patterns of health care disparities that can result, at least in part, from clinician bias, recognize disparities that are amenable to intervention and value eliminating disparities.	3, 22
21.	Describe systemic and medical-encounter issues affecting health care disparities, including communication, clinical decision-making, and patient preferences.	19

No.	Objective	Test Items
22.	Describe models of effective cross-cultural communication, assessment, and physician–patient negotiation and identify common challenges in cross-cultural communication (for example, trust, style).	34
23.	Conduct and document a culturally responsive history and physical examination within the context of family-centered care. Elicit a cultural, social, and medical history, including a patient's health beliefs and model of their illness. Demonstrate respect for a patient's cultural and health beliefs and use negotiating and problem-solving skills in shared decision-making with a patient.	9, 10, 15
24.	Describe the functions of an interpreter and effective ways of working with an interpreter. Identify when an interpreter is needed and collaborate effectively with an interpreter.	6, 7, 33
25.	Assess and enhance patient adherence based on the patient's explanatory model. Describe ways to enhance patient adherence by collaborating with traditional and other community healers.	5
26.	Critically appraise the literature as it relates to health disparities, including systems issues and quality in health care.	–
27.	Describe factors that contribute to variability in population health; outline a framework to assess communities according to population health criteria, social mores, cultural beliefs, and needs.	31
28.	Describe methods to identify key community leaders. Describe strategies for partnering with community activists to eliminate racism and other bias from health care. Develop a proposal for a community-based health intervention. Collaborate with communities to address community needs.	20

Answer Key

1. E
2. 5
3. 5
21. Disagree
22. Agree
25. Agree
30. Agree
32. D
33. F

Example of a Journal

White Memorial Medical Center
Family Medicine Residency Program

The Art of Healing

Resident Orientation Passport

This passport will be your journal to record your reflections on the selected cultural medicine activities during orientation.

1. Please answer the question(s) immediately following each session.
2. At the end of the week, you will turn in your passport to the Cultural Medicine faculty. They will read and comment on your material and return to you at the beginning of the following week.
3. To assist us in understanding your cultural knowledge, and to help us tailor future activities, passports will be collected at the end of orientation. The originals will remain with the residency, and copies can be provided to interns if requested.

> We must commit to the principle that every individual, every family, and every community has the right to receive health care services that are clinically competent, sensitive to the needs of each individual, and delivered with a sense of respect and compassion.
>
> *– Hector Flores, MD*

> We must comfort the afflicted and afflict the comfortable.
>
> *– Eleanor Roosevelt*

Passport Overview

Web-based training at thinkculturalhealth.org
- ❏ Section 1 Culturally Competent Care
- ❏ Section 2 Language Access Services
- ❏ Section 3 Organizational Supports

Family Genograms/Team Building
Cultural Medicine Workshop
- ❏ Implicit Association Test
- ❏ Doctoring in a Multicultural Society Collage
- ❏ Sorting People (Matching Faces with Races)
- ❏ Imagery Exercise
- ❏ Creative Writing Assignment
- ❏ Obstetrics/Gynecology Role Play
- ❏ Video Case Vignette (*Worlds Apart*)

Community Connections: Neighborhood Study

> There is no tolerance without respect – and no respect without knowledge.
>
> *– Professor Henry Louis Gates, Jr.*

> Cultural humility is an ongoing process that requires humility as individuals continually engage in self-reflection and self-critique, as lifelong learners and reflective practitioners.
>
> *– Melanie Tervalon, MDColor-Blindness*

> One opinion holds that ignoring race, or skin color, is the best avenue to social justice.
>
> Critics of the color-blind approach argue that it ignores research showing that, even among well-intentioned people, skin color (and other identifiable physical features such as ethnicity, gender, and physical disability) figure prominently in everyday attitudes and behavior. Thus, to get beyond racism and other similar forms of prejudice, we must first take the differences between people into account.
>
> *– American Psychological Association, 1997*

Cultural Competence

The American Medical Association defines cultural competence as 'the knowledge and interpersonal skills that allow providers to understand, appreciate and work with individuals from cultures other than their own. It involves an awareness and acceptance of cultural differences, self-awareness, knowledge of the patient's culture and adaptation of skills.'

Health Care Disparities

Disparities in the health care delivered to racial and ethnic minorities are real and are associated with worse outcomes in many cases, which is unacceptable. The real challenge lies not in debating whether disparities exist, because the evidence is overwhelming, but in developing and implementing strategies to reduce and eliminate them.

– Alan Nelson, MD

Retired physician, former president of the American Medical Association, and chair of the committee that wrote the Institute of Medicine report, *Unequal Treatment: Confronting Racial and Ethnic Disparities in Health Care* (2002).

Web-Based Cultural Curriculum and CLAS Standards (thinkculturalhealth.org)

Debriefing of Section 1: Culturally Competent Care

Describe one thing that you are committed to including in your patient care based on what you learned in this exercise and discussion.

Debriefing of Section 2: Language Access Services

Describe one thing that you are committed to including in your patient care based on what you learned in this exercise and discussion.

Debriefing of Section 3: Organizational Supports

Describe one thing that you are committed to including in your patient care practice based on what you learned in this exercise and discussion.

Family Genograms/Team Building: Your Genogram

What was it like to prepare and present your genogram?

What were some things that surprised you in either the preparation or presentation process? Describe at least two.

Family Genograms/Team Building: Others' Genogram

What was it like to listen to colleagues' presentations? What will you carry with you from this exercise? Complete an entry for each of the three sessions.

Session 1:

Session 2:

Session 3:

ACTIVITY 1 Cultural Medicine Workshop

Implicit Association Test – Gender and Sexual Orientation

What did you observe about your performance?

How does this new information inform your role of physician?

If your performance is typical of physicians, how might this impact quality of care and health care disparities?

Doctoring in a Multicultural Society Collage

What reaction did you have when you saw the completed collage? (Complete question in debriefing session.)

Discuss two challenges and two opportunities of increasing diversity in health care.

ACTIVITY 3 Cultural Medicine Workshop

Sorting People (Matching Faces with Races)

The most important thing I learned about my perceptions of race was . . .

Tell a story about how you felt when one of your physical characteristics (gender, height, weight, features, skin color, etc.) led to stereotyping by someone.

What will you do differently in meeting and assessing patients after completing this exercise?

ACTIVITY 4 Cultural Medicine Workshop

Imagery Exercise

Describe at least one of your stereotypes that you discovered in this exercise.

Describe at least two ways your own attitudes and stereotypes might affect the quality of the patient care you provide.

ACTIVITY 5 Cultural Medicine Workshop

Creative Writing Assignment

Read the poem *Maria* by R. Campo aloud twice and then, with the patient's voice, write about this doctor–patient encounter.

What physician biases do you detect in the poem?

Describe two ways your own biases or attitudes might affect your cross-cultural communication with patients?

ACTIVITY 6 Cultural Medicine Workshop

Obstetrics/Gynecology Role Play

How are you going to work with patients with attitudes different from your own regarding obstetrical/gynecological care?

What beliefs do you hold that might conflict with those of patients in our community? Describe one that relates directly to decision-making in regards to the care of patients.

ACTIVITY 7 Cultural Medicine Workshop

Video Case Vignette (*Worlds Apart*)

The case provided cross-cultural challenges to communication and effective care of Justine Chitsena. Describe three of the challenges illustrated in this case.

What was your impression of the negotiation between the family and the medical staff?

Describe the role you intend negotiation will play in your care of patients here at WMMC.

Community Connections: Neighborhood Study

Describe what you learned from participating in the neighborhood study and creating your map.

Describe three things you learned about this community from the presentations of the other two groups.

Name: _____(Back Cover)

Date: _____

Faculty Signature/Passport Stamp

Web-based Training 1 _____

Web-based Training 2 _____

Web-based Training 3 _____

Family Genograms 1 _____

Family Genograms 2 _____

Family Genograms 3 _____

Cultural Medicine Workshop _____

Community Connections: Neighborhood Study _____

Cultural Competence SOAP Grid

The clinical encounter between clinician and patient is where the skills of a culturally responsive provider are put to the greatest test. As such, the discussion of patient cases and doctor–patient encounters in precepting sessions and in inpatient rounds provides an excellent opportunity for raising culturally relevant issues to enhance learning and to assess learners.

The SOAP Grid was designed to offer faculty instructors a number of 'onramps' to discussion of cultural issues in a typical case presentation. The body of the grid is comprised of specific questions for the resident/student regarding the subjective, objective, assessment, and plan components of a case. There is also an additional row entitled 'Post-Hoc Reflection' that provides a number of 'big picture' follow-up questions about culture and patient care.

For the horizontal axis of the grid, we selected three thematic areas which merit attention in caring for culturally diverse patients:
1. the degree to which this case reflects, or might become an instance of, a health disparity or inequitable care;
2. the degree to which medical errors are possible and can be prevented in the provision of care to this patient;
3. the degree to which the intervention is reflective of a patient-centered care model of doctoring.

This is a starting point. We hope that preceptors will use the grid to guide their inquiries to help learners become accustomed to regularly considering these issues as they care for patients, and to enhance their development as culturally responsive clinicians.

Subjective Components of a Case

	Health Disparities	Medical Errors	Patient-Oriented Care
Subjective	Did patient self-identify gender, race, age, ethnicity, marital status, sexual orientation, etc.? If not, how did you determine the patient's demographics? Considering evidence-based medical literature, is the patient empirically at risk for any health disparities?	Any missing data due to assumptions made? Think about your life context in comparison to that of the patient. Any blind spots? Did you encounter any language issues? How did you handle them? Did the patient appear distrustful of the health care system? Were you able to establish a relationship of trust with the patient? If not, what next?	Did you ask about the patient's health beliefs (Q2)? What parts of the patient's story require follow up in the next visit?

Health Disparities

These questions guide the learner to look at their patient in new ways. The learner is asked to take the 'race/ethnicity' question seriously, and to check any incorrect assumptions about the patient they may have made if they have not asked the patient for a self-reported description of ethnicity, age, gender, etc. Right up front, the preceptor turns the resident's attention to health disparity risk factors, given the demographic information collected. With this information, the learner is encouraged to form hypotheses and consider the patient in a greater context of empirically based health risk factors. Example: did you consider anemia in this African-American well-child visit? (One fifth to one third of Black children are anemic.)

Medical Errors

With these questions, the preceptor helps the learner to increase the validity of the data being collected in two ways. First, the dyad addresses any past experience or negative outcome that might influence the patient's trust in the medical system. The resident/student is also asked to consider his/her own life context and possible unrecognized assumptions. The resident is then asked to consider his/her role in establishing and deepening trust in the clinician–patient relationship. Second, language issues and proper use of interpreters, as necessary, can be directly addressed.

Patient-Oriented Care

With these questions, the preceptor helps the learner consider the degree to which the patient's views and perceptions are embraced and considered in the doctor–patient relationship and data collection portions of the visit. This data will provide an important base for later treatment plan negotiations. Clearly, a doctor–patient relationship evolves over time. It can be instructive for the learner to consider what information, background, cultural beliefs, and world view information they plan to explore in future visits.

Objective Components of a Case

	Health Disparities	Medical Errors	Patient-Oriented Care
Objective	Does your exam and lab data address all of the patient's disparity risks (e.g. BMI for overweight patients)?	Did you defer, delay, or eliminate any aspect of the physical exam for reasons of your discomfort or patient refusal (e.g. for cultural, religious, gender preferences)? What should your next step be?	Did you feel uncomfortable at any time while conducting the physical exam? How did it impact the exam? What should you do to grow from this experience? Did the patient appear uncomfortable during your exam? If so, how did you address the patient's feelings?

Health Disparities

The inquiry here builds on the subjective data, now assessing the completeness, appropriateness, and focus of the physical exam in the context of the patient's demographics and empirically based probabilities of becoming a health disparity statistic. The preceptor might also inquire into the cultural respectfulness employed by the learner in conducting the physical exam. Example: what objective data should you collect on this African-American child to determine if anemia is a problem?

Medical Errors

Here the learner is asked to examine the completeness of the physical exam. A number of variables can intervene, which can lead to shortcuts or less-than-complete examinations. The comfort level of the physician with individual patients (or 'certain types' of patients) is a topic of great importance for discussion and reflection, despite the discomfort such discussions can raise for both learners and faculty members. Furthermore, the learner is asked to consider how to handle patient refusals regarding necessary exam components. The key here is to avoid medical errors by directly addressing difficult issues. Example: a Muslim male patient that does not want a female physician to conduct the genitourinary exam.

Patient-Oriented Care

When a physician is uncomfortable with some aspect of the patient or the physical examination process, there is a risk of incomplete or substandard care. Similarly, when a patient is uncomfortable with an aspect of the physical examination or feels that the provider has violated a cultural boundary, data is lost and the provider–patient relationship is jeopardized. Example: potential incomplete examination of an angry patient or a smelly patient.

Assessment Components of a Case

	Health Disparities	Medical Errors	Patient-Oriented Care
Assessment	How does your assessment address cultural differences in disease manifestation? How have you considered any 'problems behind the current medical issue' related to the patient's life context (e.g. homelessness, abuse, poverty, family, substance use)?	Have you made any untested assumptions about this patient that will influence your differential diagnosis or final assessment?	In your assessment/problem list, do you address the patient's reasons for coming to the clinic? Does the patient understand and agree with your assessment, and how do you know? Are there any discrepancies between your assessment and the patient's health belief system? Please describe.

Health Disparities

Here preceptors focus in on culturally responsive differential diagnosis and unique presentations of illness across groups. Furthermore, the learner is encouraged to consider the patient's medical issues in the context of their life, including the socio-cultural, familial, psychological, economic, environmental, legal, political, and spiritual aspects. Example: if this child is anemic, what issues within the context of his/her life should be examined to determine the root cause?

Medical Errors

Here the preceptor can offer the resident another opportunity for reflection on the case at hand, with a focus on the validity of assumptions, and/or the undue influences of unconscious biases or stereotypes. The focus is on accuracy of assessment and diagnosis to ensure correct care and prevent errors that can result in harm.

Patient-Oriented Care

These questions help the learner approach the treatment planning stage with a patient-centered mindset that includes a negotiated, mutually agreeable strategy to address the presenting complaints. Patients who are uncomfortable with an aspect of a treatment plan, or who feel that a personal belief or boundary has been violated, are less likely to adhere to the treatment plan, much less return to the same provider. These questions help the learner consider and attempt to rectify any such problems in the clinical encounter. Preceptors may also encourage learners to directly explore and address provider–patient discrepancies in the assessment of the problem, as a central tenant of patient-centered care.

Plan Components of a Case

	Health Disparities	Medical Errors	Patient-Oriented Care
Plan	How have you used knowledge of health disparities in creating your plan?	Is anything omitted from your plan based on 'who' this patient is (e.g. likeable, deserving, etc)?	Any concerns about the patient's ability or willingness to adhere to the treatment plan, and how did you negotiate issues with the patient?
	How did you insure that the patient is able and willing to adhere to the plan, within his/her life context?	Did you encounter any literacy or language issues? How did you handle them?	How did you address any patient concerns regarding potential adverse effects of your treatment plan?

Health Disparities

The questions in this category aim to insure that unconscious racial bias (*see* Schulman KA, Berlin JA, Harless W, 1999) type errors are avoided in this very important treatment-planning stage of care. Learners are encouraged to use their knowledge related to evidence-based medicine and health disparities to develop an optimal plan. They are also encouraged to ensure that the plan is appropriate for the patient within the context of his/her life, and will thus encourage adherence. Example: considering the child's life context, how should the anemia be addressed to help ensure both short-term and long-term health?

Medical Errors

Learners are encouraged to reconsider the completeness of their treatment plan, and to identify any patient characteristics or doctor–patient dynamics that may have interfered. This is also an opportunity to reflect on any language or communication issues that may have emerged to the detriment of care provided. A forthright review of a treatment plan with harm reduction in mind can forestall medical errors and untoward consequences of care. Example: offering birth control methods to a female lesbian patient would be a failure of respect and understanding.

Patient-Oriented Care

The questions in this category strike right at the heart of negotiated care, embracing the patient's world views and health beliefs. Learners should be encouraged to explore potential treatment adherence barriers with the patient, as well as evaluate the degree to which the patient fully understands and 'buys in' to the treatment regimen.

Post-Hoc Reflections of a Case

	Health Disparities	Medical Errors	Patient-Oriented Care
Post-Hoc Reflection	Was there a health care disparity already affecting the patient's health status prior to the patient visit? How did the assessment and plan change based on the discussion of health disparities? How can we avoid health disparities for future patients?	What are the special communication needs of our patient? Do any require follow-up with other health care providers? Are we at risk for poor outcomes based on patient's health practices (e.g. complementary and alternative medication)?	What is your plan to become more knowledgeable and skillful in regard to this patient's special population? What went well and what did not work in your negotiation with this patient? How can models with acronyms like ETHNIC and LEARN assist you in your care of patients?

Health Disparities

Here the learner is asked to engage in a brief practice-based learning and improvement exercise. The learner is asked to consider pre-existing health disparities, how his/her own assessment and plan has changed based on discussion with their preceptor, and how the clinic/hospital can avoid contributing to future health disparities. Example: what other problems, common to African-American children, should you be considering when conducting a well-child visit?

Medical Errors

These post-hoc reflection questions ask the learner to explore beyond this case to the systems based practice issues, e.g. communication with other providers and complementary and alternative care.

Patient-Oriented Care

Learners are asked to consider goals for future learning regarding cultural knowledge and negotiation strategies raised by this case. They will only become proficient in negotiating treatment plans if they are instructed, supported, and later reflect on negotiations so as to glean new learning that can be applied to future patients. The learner will not always feel completely at ease with negotiated treatment plans, and may require modeling and tangible instruction as to how to maximize their success in achieving true doctor–patient collaboration. Models with acronyms like ETHNIC and LEARN may be of assistance to some learners.

Multi-Station Cultural Examination or Multi-Station Teaching Exercise Potential Stations

	Sample Stations	Curriculum Objectives	Competency Assessed
1.	Go the PBS Race website and click on 'Sorting People': http://www.pbs.org/race/002_SortingPeople/002_00-home.htm. Complete the exercise. Read the section on 'What is Race?' (10 Facts about Race.) Write a paragraph describing your definition of race and ethnicity based on what you learned on the website.	1	Knowledge
2.	Review the following list: cultural heritage, gender, class, ethnic-racial identity, sexual orientation, disability, and spirituality. 1. Select one area and discuss the health risks and protective factors you have derived from that element of your culture. 2. Select a second area and list the benefits and detriments to you so far in your life regarding your status within the category (e.g. female, Jewish, Russian, etc.).	2	Awareness and knowledge
3.	Go to the PBS Race website and click on 'Human Diversity': http://www.pbs.org/race/004_HumanDiversity/004_00-home.htm Take the quiz. 1. Describe what you learned about race and human diversity. 2. Make a table with two columns entitled 'challenges' and 'opportunities'. Complete the two lists in relation to the increasing diversity among health care providers.	3	Attitude and knowledge
4.	Written exercise: list the benefits and challenges of increased diversity in patients and the benefits and challenges of increased diversity in providers. Select one benefit and one challenge and discuss.	3	Knowledge
5.	Complete the Implicit Association Test for Arabs and answer these questions. 1. What did you learn about your potential for bias and stereotyping either from the exercise or its results? 2. Describe how unintentional bias might affect clinical decision-making.	4	Awareness and knowledge
6.	Go to the PBS Race website 'Me My Race and I' and view the clip *Split Identity*: http://www.pbs.org/race/005_MeMyRaceAndI/005_00-home.htm 1. Write a paragraph describing your reactions to the clip. 2. Discuss how these kinds of perceptions might impact patient presentation and physician/provider clinical decision-making in your clinical site.	6	Attitude
7.	Go to the PBS Race website 'Me My Race and I' and view the clip *The Elephant in the Room*: http://www.pbs.org/race/005_MeMyRaceAndI/005_00-home.htm 1. Write a paragraph describing your reactions to the clip. 2. Describe one thing you can do right now to help reduce your biases and those of other health care providers.	7	Attitude
8.	Review the 'Highlights' for the most recent *National Health Care Disparities Report* and examine the progress for non-White Hispanics and poor people as described in the report. 1. Discuss how well the country is doing in quality versus access for these two groups. 2. Select an area of disparity where clinician bias could be contributing. Describe one thing you can do to help address the problem.	8, 14	Application of knowledge
9.	Review the 'Highlights' for the most recent *National Health Care Quality Report* and examine the progress for settings of care and phase of care. 1. Discuss progress by setting and phase of care (best, worst). 2. Select one area of challenge (within setting or phase of care) and list three ways you could help address the problem.	8, 14	Application of knowledge
10.	Review the most recent California *County Health Status Profiles* and examine how your county compares to the California average and to the *Healthy People 2010* goals. 1. List three areas where your county falls below the *Healthy People 2010* goals. 2. Explore these areas further by examining the *California Death Rates by Zip Code Report*. 3. Discuss how your clinic/hospital's zip code compares to the overall county data. 4. Select one area and list a) underlying causes (e.g. social determinants) for each area and b) barriers to addressing disparities.	9, 11, 13	Application of knowledge

cont.

	Sample Stations	Curriculum Objectives	Competency Assessed
11.	Review the most recent *National Health Care Disparities Report* and examine the progress for either African-Americans or non-White Hispanics in the area of diabetes. 1. Discuss areas of challenge. 2. List underlying causes for disparity for your patient population including social determinants, health beliefs, and culturally related risk and protective factors. 3. Describe how you might partner with community leaders to address these challenges.	8, 24, 25	Application of knowledge
12.	Go to the PBS Race website 'Me My Race and I' and view the clip *To See or Not to See*: http://www.pbs.org/race/005_MeMyRaceAndI/005_00-home.htm 1. Write a paragraph describing your reactions to the clip. 2. Describe how historical, political, environmental, and institutional factors might impact health and underlie health care disparities.	10	Application of knowledge
13.	Written exercise. 1. (5 minutes) From your own patient contact experience and those of your peers, list as many specific health beliefs (culturally/historically based) as you can remember in relation to a) maintaining health, b) care during pregnancy/delivery, c) end-of-life rituals. 2. (10 minutes) Describe one mnemonic or model that you can use to gather these types of data from your patients.	17, 18	Application of knowledge
14.	Standardized Patient Exercise. Conduct an interview to discern the patient's current concerns, underlying healing tradition and health beliefs in relation to their health problem(s). (Rated by patient or observer.)	17, 18, 21	Skill
15.	View the Kaiser video clip *Sickle cell crisis in the ER*. 1. What role, if any, did race, ethnicity, or culture play in this encounter? 2. Discuss how the inherent power imbalance between provider and patient impacted the result. 3. Discuss how you might prevent this happening at our institution.	19, 20	Application of knowledge
16.	Standardized Patient Exercise. Conduct a culturally responsive history and physical exam of a patient from another culture with abdominal pain. (Rated by patient or observer.)	21	Skill
17.	Standardized Patient Exercise. Conduct a culturally responsive history with a patient who speaks another language using the telephonic interpretation system. (Rated by patient or observer.)	22	Skill

Primer on Multi-Station Examinations (OSCE/OSCA/CSA/PBA/CPX)

Julie G. Nyquist, PhD (reprinted with permission from author)

Introduction
The multi-station clinical examination has become an established technique that continues to experience increasing use in the overall assessment of learner clinical performance.

Advantages
❏ Standardized administration.
❏ Potentially good reliability.
❏ Can provide excellent individual feedback from expert clinicians.

Disadvantages
❏ Expensive to prepare and administer.
❏ Educational and clinical experts need to work together.
❏ Can be logistically difficult to administer.

In the multi-station clinical examination, students rotate through a series of stations and undertake a wide variety of clinically related tasks. Each station is designed to assess specific clinical, interpersonal, or technical skills, or some aspect of problem solving. Stations vary in design, complexity, and amount of time needed. Multiple station exams with brief stations, 5–10 minutes per station, are often called an Objective Structured Clinical Examination/Assessment or OSCE/OSCA. These exams focus on assessment of individual skills and performance components. Examples of typical station tasks include:
❏ read and interpret a radiograph;
❏ read and interpret a microscope slide;
❏ give a limited physical exam to a real patient;
❏ take a drug and alcohol history from a standardized patient;
❏ discuss a Do Not Resuscitate order with an actor in the role of a family member;
❏ speak on the telephone with a standardized patient in the role of a parent needing immediate advice about a child's illness.

Multiple station exams with longer stations, 15–30 minutes per station, are often called a Clinical Skills Assessment (CSA), Performance-Based Assessments/Examinations (PBA/PBX) or occasionally, Clinical Performance Examinations (CPX). In this type of assessment, the focus is on assessment of the overall practitioner-patient encounter and the tasks are more integrated, often including both the relevant history and physical examination, or both of these plus an interview and provision of relevant counseling. Typical tasks include:
❏ conduct a focused history and physical exam for a patient presenting with abdominal pain;
❏ take a relevant history from a patient presenting with persistent fever;
❏ conduct of a pregnancy risk assessment;
❏ conduct an HIV risk assessment and provide pretest counseling;
❏ provide bad news to a patient about some disease;
❏ provide preventive advice to a teenager.

Some multi-station exams use the standardized patient as the evaluator, some use practitioner observers, while some require a written response which is later scored by a practitioner. Data gathered at stations involving patients is almost always recorded on rating scales, carefully developed for the specific behaviors to be assessed. In addition, some exams also include inter-station activities that focus on assessment of problem solving or assessment of relevant knowledge. Several things must happen for this method to be successful. First, educational and clinical experts must work together to develop a truly effective examination. Second, initial research evidence indicates that from 8–18 stations are needed for a reliable evaluation. Finally, assessing a large number of students in this manner is logistically difficult, and requires a team of people.

What Criteria? How Will Pass/Fail Be Determined?

1. Pass/fail can be based on normative performance or criterion-referenced performance.
   - Normative: cut point generally set between 1.5 and 2.0 standard deviations below the mean. Passing depends on how well a student did in comparison to other students.
   - Criterion referenced: based on how well each student did in comparison to some standard, generally set at a percent of total score or percent of all stations passed.
2. If pass/fail is based on comparison to a standard (criterion referenced), performance may be based on:
   - percent of total points achieved on entire test (compensatory model; very high performance on some stations can offset low performance on others); or
   - percent of all stations passed.
3. If pass/fail is criterion referenced, will stations which are very difficult (less than 30–40% of students passing) be modified or omitted from scoring?

How Will Data Collection and Analysis Be Done? Who is Responsible and What Kinds of Analysis Will Be Done?

1. Data collection: logistics for test need to be arranged.
   a) A station coordinator (in charge of station development and administration) needs to be selected for each station and monitored to be certain that:
      - specific case content and tasks are selected;
      - written case materials and rating forms are developed;
      - materials and supplies needed for station are specified in advance;
      - if required – real patient or standardized patient selected and trained;
      - raters are selected and trained (and show up at their assigned times for testing).
   b) Clerical support needs to be obtained to ensure that:
      —all materials needed for each station (tongue depressors, sterile gloves, x-ray viewers, microscopes, etc.) are in examination area on day(s) of test;
      —all rating forms and other materials are copied in sufficient numbers and are available in examination area on day(s) of test;
      —learners are assigned times to be tested, notified of those times, and provided with appropriate instructions about what will happen;
      —rotation schedules, time sheets, site and station maps, etc. for each testing session are created and available in examination area on day(s) of test;
      —general instructions to all participants are written and distributed – these include when and where to come, and the duties for each group (raters, patients, students).
2. Decision needs to be made concerning how analysis will be done.
   - Consider the decisions made above related to how test will be scored.
   - Include results by student and by station to facilitate good feedback.
   - Include item analysis for each station to facilitate good *post hoc* review.

Feedback and Action – Who Will Receive Feedback and What Actions Will Be Taken Related to Poor/Inadequate Student Performance?

1. Feedback: there needs to be a mechanism for providing feedback that ensures timely and meaningful feedback to students, administrators, test and station coordinators, and raters.
2. Action: what happens to students who perform poorly needs to be decided in advance.
   - Opportunities for remediation should be determined.
   - Summative consequences, if any, should be decided.
3. *Post hoc* review: post-administration review by the test and station coordinators should include:
   - reflection on examination process;
   - subjective and objective review of examination results for purposes of:
      —examining individual student performance;
      —examining overall group performance;
      —looking for strengths/weaknesses in curriculum;

—examination of station-by-station results to see how station and rating form worked;

—review of each rating form using the item analysis.

Multi-Station Clinical Examination Station-Specific Decisions

Determination of Specific Station Content and Station Tasks

Content of individual stations should be:

❏ consistent with the test plan for the overall multi-station clinical examination;

❏ common and important to general medicine;

❏ something you would want every graduate to be able to accomplish.

Determination About How Performance in Each Station Will Be Rated

1. Develop a systematic rating procedure for each station.
   a) Determine type of score to be used.
      —Percent of points is the easiest method since each station can have a different number of raw score points.
      —Forcing all stations to have the same number of raw score points can be very awkward.
      —Better to award points for things done correctly; subtracting points can result in a negative score for some examinees – this is not helpful. Also, subtracting points does not add to reliability of scoring.
   b) Determine who will observe, faculty (choose which ones) or trained patient.
   c) Develop rating forms: important aspects of the skill should be rated on a specially designed form. Given the short time allotted, a rating scale of no more than three categories (e.g. performed correctly, performed partially, performed incorrectly or omitted) is appropriate.
   d) Train observers.
      —Orient raters to the specific criteria.
      —If possible, practice using the form before it is put into use.
   e) Set standards: generally should be set as part of overall test plan.
2. If feedback is to be provided in the station, determine type of feedback and prepare raters to give helpful feedback.

Preparation of the Actual Station

1. Select and modify station.
   a) Approval of content area.
   b) Design/approval of rating form.
   c) Design/approval of written test material.
   d) Ensure that task fits within station time limit.
2. Gather/prepare materials and supplies needed.
   a) Machinery such as x-ray viewer, microscope, etc.
   b) Supplies, such as cotton swabs, sterile gloves, etc.
   c) Patients, either actual or simulated (provide training as required).
3. Prepare examination administration.
   a) Select raters for station.
   b) Train raters on checklist or rating scale devised.

Post-Administration Review of Station Results

Review of station results is important for improvement of the station in future tests and for overall improvement of the test itself. An item analysis (including item difficulty and some measure of item discrimination) should be used to help examine the effectiveness of the rating form.

Resources

Carraccio C, Englander R. The objective-structured clinical examination: a step in the direction of competency-based evaluation. *Arch Pediatr Adolesc Med*. 2000; **154**(7): 736–41.

Colliver JA, Swartz MH. Assessing clinical performance with standardized patients. *JAMA*. 1997; **278**: 790–1.

Goff BA, Lentz GM, Lee D, *et al*. Development of an objective structured assessment of technical skills for obstetric and gynecology residents. *Obstet Gynecol*. 2000; **96**(1): 146–50.

Harden RM, Stevenson M, Downie WW, *et al*. Assessment of clinical competence using objective structured examination. *BMJ*. 1975; **1**: 447–51.

Hodges B, Turnbull J, Cohen R, *et al*. Evaluating communication skills in the OSCE format: reliability and generalizability. *Med Educ*. 1996; **30**: 38–43.

Humphrey-Murto S, Smee S, Touchie C, *et al*. A comparison of physician examiners and trained assessors in a high-stakes OSCE setting. *Acad Med*. 2005 Oct; **80**(10 Suppl.): S59–62.

Humphris GM, Kaney S. The objective structured video exam for assessment of communication skills. *Med Educ*. 2000; **34**: 939–45.

Junger J, Schafer S, Roth C, *et al*. Effects of basic clinical skills training on objective structured clinical examination performance. *Med Educ*. 2005 Oct; **39**(10): 1015–20.

Keely E, Myers K, Dojeiji S. Can written communication skills be tested in an objective structured clinical examination format? *Acad Med*. 2002; **77**: 82–6.

McLaughlin K, Gregor L, Jones A, *et al*. Can standardized patients replace physicians as OSCE examiners? *BMC Med Educ*. 2006; **6**: 12.

Prislin MD, Fitzpatrick CF, Lie D, *et al*. Use of an objective structured clinical examination in evaluating student performance. *Fam Med*. 1998; **30**: 338–44.

Reznick R, Regehr G, MacRae H, *et al*. Testing technical skill via an innovative "bench station" examination. *Am J Surg*. 1997; **173**: 226–30.

Roberts C, Wass V, Jones R, *et al*. A discourse analysis study of 'good' and 'poor' communication in an OSCE: a proposed new framework for teaching students. *Med Educ*. 2003; **37**(3): 192–201.

Schoonheim-Klein M. Walmsley AD, Habets L, *et al*. An implementation strategy for introducing an OSCE into a dental school. *Eur J Dent Educ*. 2005 Nov; **9**(4): 143–9.

Sultana CJ. The objective structured assessment of technical skills and the ACGME competencies. *Obstet Gynecol Clin North Am*. 2006 Jun; **33**(2): 259–65, viii.

van der Vleuten CPM, Swanson DB. Assessment of clinical skills with standardized patients: state of the art. *Teach Learn Med*. 1990; **2**: 58–76.

Walters K, Osborn D, Raven P. The development, validity and reliability of a multimodality objective structured clinical examination in psychiatry. *Med Educ*. 2005; **39**(3): 292–8.

Wass V, Roberts C, Hoogenboom R, *et al*. Effect of ethnicity on performance in a final objective structured clinical examination: qualitative and quantitative study. *BMJ*. 2003; **326**(7393): 800–3.

Yudkowsky R, Alseidi A, Cintron J. Beyond fulfilling the core competencies: an objective structured clinical examination to assess communication and interpersonal skills in a surgical residency. *Curr Surg*. 2004 Sep–Oct; **61**(5): 499–503.

Sample Commitment to Change

Name:_____ Date: _____

Session: Contributors to Health Disparities
Reminders:
1. Definition of disparity: 'the differences in the incidence, prevalence, mortality, and burden of disease and other adverse health conditions that exist among specific population groups in the United States' (source: National Institutes of Health).
2. Contributors to health disparities: person, providers, health care system and society.

Describe the primary lesson you learned in this session:

List two things that you will do differently as a physician in your professional life based on what you learned in this session:
1.

2.

Cultural Competence Precepting Questionnaire

Directions

Please answer the following questions in relation to your precepting activities with learners during 1. your time teaching in the inpatient service; and 2. while precepting in the ambulatory care center. Check the column that most closely reflects the frequency with which you do each activity.

Activities		Check One Column			
1. During a typical month of precepting on the inpatient service, how often do you ask a resident or discuss with a resident each of the following:		Daily	Once a week	Once a month	Never
a)	The context of a patient's life (story, personal situation, culture, family, etc.)?				
b)	Patient's health beliefs (what a patient thought made them ill and what might make them better)?				
c)	Use of complementary provider or traditional healers?				
d)	Scientific evidence for recommended treatments?				
e)	Treatment in the context of evidence merged with health beliefs?				
f)	Proper negotiation of post-discharge care with a patient?				
2. During a typical month of precepting in the Family Health Center, how often to you ask a resident or discuss with a resident each of the following:		Daily	Once a week	Once a month	Never
a)	The context of a patient's life (story, personal situation, family, etc.)?				
b)	Patient's health beliefs (what a patient thought made them ill and what might make them better)?				
c)	Use of complementary provider or traditional healers?				
d)	Scientific evidence for the diagnosis or care plan?				
e)	Treatment in the context of evidence merged with health beliefs?				
f)	Proper negotiation of care with a patient?				

Approximately how many months per year do you teach in the inpatient setting?

Approximately how many months per year do you teach in the ambulatory care center?

Comments:

Sample Cultural Competence Training Questionnaire

	Cultural Competence Curriculum	Orientation Month	Continuity Clinic	Behavioral Science – Community Medicine	Inpatient Rotations	Outpatient Rotations	Adolescent Medicine	Hospice/Geriatrics

Directions: for each item below, check where you have gained relevant attitudes/appreciation, knowledge, skills or behaviors. Check all that apply.

If you have not participated in any rotation/activity, mark the NA (not applicable) column in the first row.

NA – Check in this row any activity not yet experienced.

1. Define race, ethnicity, and culture.

2. Become aware of own cultural heritage and life context and describe it.

3. Value the importance of diversity in health care.

4. Discuss patterns of national data on health, health care disparities, and quality of health care.

5. Discuss of health and health care disparities in the local community using *Healthy People 2010* and other resources.

6. Value the importance of social determinants and community factors on health and strive to prevent disparities.

7. Describe historical models of health beliefs and the questions about health practices important in the local community.

8a. Identify healing traditions and beliefs of patients and/or their families, including ethno-medical beliefs and use of ethno-medical healers.

8b. Elicit patient preferences; listen and respond appropriately to patient feedback about key cross-cultural issues.

9. Discuss race, ethnicity, and culture in the context of the medical interview and health care. Exhibit comfort when conversing with patients/colleagues about cultural issues.

10. Recognize and describe institutional cultural issues for own institution.

11. Value the importance of curiosity, empathy, and respect in patient care and the importance of continuous growth as a healer.

12. Recognize own potential for bias and stereotyping, be able to identify own stereotypes and biases and explore how attitudes, biases, and stereotypes affect clinical encounters, clinical decision-making and quality of care.

13. Identify and appreciate how clinician bias and stereotyping can affect interactions with patients, families, communities, and other members of the health care team, and the link between effective communication and quality care.

14. Describe the impact of the patient's context (cultural heritage, gender, class, ethnic-racial identity, sexual orientation, disability, age, and spirituality) on clinical decision-making.

cont.

	Cultural Competence Curriculum	Orientation Month	Continuity Clinic	Behavioral Science – Community Medicine	Inpatient Rotations	Outpatient Rotations	Adolescent Medicine	Hospice/Geriatrics

Directions: for each item below, check where you have gained relevant attitudes/appreciation, knowledge, skills or behaviors. Check all that apply.

If you have not participated in any rotation/activity, mark the NA (not applicable) column in the first row.

15. Describe strategies for reducing physician's own biases, and those of others and demonstrate strategies to assess, manage, and reduce bias and its effects in the clinical encounter and in clinical practice.

16. Describe the inherent power imbalance between physician and patient and how it affects the clinical encounter.

17. Recognize and describe how access, historical, political, environmental, and institutional factors (including racism and discrimination) impact health and underlie health and health care disparities.

18. Identify how race, ethnicity and social determinants of health (e.g., education, culture, socioeconomic status, housing and employment) affect health and health care quality, cost, and outcomes.

19. Identify and discuss the contributors to disparities (patient, provider, health care system and society) and discuss the challenges and barriers to eliminating health disparities.

20. Describe patterns of health care disparities that can result, at least in part, from clinician bias, recognize disparities that are amenable to intervention and value eliminating disparities.

21. Describe systemic and medical-encounter issues related to health care disparities, including communication issues, clinical decision-making, and patient preferences.

22. Describe models of effective cross-cultural communication, assessment, and physician–patient negotiation and identify common challenges in cross-cultural communication (e.g. trust, style).

23. Conduct and document a culturally responsive history and physical examination within the context of family-centered care. Elicit a cultural, social, and medical history, including a patient's health beliefs/model of their illness. Demonstrate respect for patients' cultural and health beliefs and use negotiating and problem-solving skills in shared decision-making with a patient.

24. Describe the functions of an interpreter and effective ways of working with an interpreter. Identify when an interpreter is needed and collaborate effectively with an interpreter.

25. Assess and enhance patient adherence based on the patient's explanatory model. Describe ways to enhance patient adherence by collaborating with traditional/community healers.

26. Critically appraise literature relating to health disparities, including systems issues and quality in health care.

27. Describe how to assess a community or specific population in relation to health criteria, social mores, and cultural beliefs.

28. Describe strategies for partnering with the local community and collaborate to address community needs.

Evaluation References

Aeder L, Altshuler L, Kachur E, *et al*. The 'Culture OSCE': introducing a formative assessment into a postgraduate program. *Educ Health*. 2007 May; **20**(1): 11.

Assemi M, Cullander C, Hudmon KS. Psychometric analysis of a scale assessing self-efficacy for cultural competence in patient counseling. *Ann Pharmacother*. 2006 Dec; **40**(12): 2130–5.

Brathwaite AC, Majumdar B. Evaluation of a cultural competence educational programme. *J Adv Nurs*. 2006; **53**(4): 470–9.

Ciesielka DJ, Schumacher G, Conway A, *et al*. Implementing and evaluating a culturally-focused curriculum in a collaborative graduate nursing program. *Int J Nurs Educ Scholarsh*. 2005; **2**: Article 6.

Crisp C. The Gay Affirmative Practice Scale (GAP): a new measure for assessing cultural competence with gay and lesbian clients. *Soc Work*. 2006 Apr; **51**(2): 115–26.

Crosson JC, Deng W, Brazeau C, *et al*. Evaluating the effect of cultural competency training on medical student attitudes. *Fam Med*. 2004 Mar; **36**(3): 199–203.

Doorenbos AZ, Schim SM, Benkert R, *et al*. Psychometric evaluation of the cultural competence assessment instrument among healthcare providers. *Nurs Res*. 2005 Sep–Oct; **54**(5): 324–31.

Gordon J. Assessing students' personal and professional development using portfolios and interviews. *Med Educ*. 2003; **37**(4): 335–40.

Ladson GM, Lin JM, Flores A, *et al*. An assessment of cultural competence of first- and second-year medical students at a historically diverse medical school. *Am J Obstet Gynecol*. 2006 Nov; **195**(5): 1457–62.

Lie D, Boker J, Cleveland E. Using the tool for assessing cultural competence training (TACCT) to measure faculty and medical student perceptions of cultural competence instruction in the first three years of the curriculum. *Acad Med*. 2006 Jun; **81**(6): 557–64.

Miller E, Green AR. Student reflections on learning cross-cultural skills through a 'cultural competence' OSCE. *Med Teach*. 2007 May; **29**(4): e76–84.

Peña Dolhun E, Muñoz C, Grumbach K. Cross-cultural education in U.S. medical schools: development of an assessment tool. *Acad Med*. 2003 Jun; **78**(6): 615–22.

Price EG, Beach MC, Gary TL, *et al*. A systematic review of the methodological rigor of studies evaluating cultural competence training of health professionals. *Acad Med*. 2005 Jun; **80**(6): 578–86.

Rowland ML, Bean CY, Casamassimo PS. A snapshot of cultural competency education in US dental schools. *J Dent Educ*. 2006 Sep; **70**(9): 982–90.

Rutledge CM, Garzon L, Scott M, *et al*. Using standardized patients to teach and evaluate nurse practitioner students on cultural competency. *Int J Nurs Educ Scholarsh*. 2004; **1**: Article 17.

Schim SM, Doorenbos AZ, Miller J, *et al*. Development of a cultural competence assessment instrument. *J Nurs Meas*. 2003 Spring–Summer; **11**(1): 29–40.

Selig S, Tropiano E, Greene-Moton E. Teaching cultural competence to reduce health disparities. *Health Promot Pract*. 2006 Jul; **7**(3 Suppl.): 247S–55S.

Shapiro J, Hollingshead J, Morrison E. Self-perceived attitudes and skills of cultural competence: a comparison of family medicine and internal medicine residents. *Med Teach*. 2003 May; **25**(3): 327–9.

Siegel C, Haugland G, Chambers ED. Performance measures and their benchmarks for assessing organizational cultural competency in behavioral health care service delivery. *Adm Policy Ment Health*. 2003 Nov; **31**(2): 141–70.

Stanhope V, Solomon P, Pernell-Arnold A, *et al*. Evaluating cultural competence among behavioral health professionals. *Psychiatr Rehab J*. 2005; **28**(3): 225–33.

Section 7

Resources and References

Resources and References:
Overview and Table of Contents

Overview

In this section you will find listings of resources in four categories: web-based resources, video resources, reference books, and journal articles. The resource listings are not intended to be exhaustive. The listings are meant to include all materials used in preparation of the curriculum. Most resources are cited in Section 3, Section 4, and Section 5.

Table of Contents

Web-Based Resources

Overview
The web resources section includes resources we used in preparing the curriculum. It is divided into seven sections by types of content.
1. Health disparities and diversity: sites that provide reports and/or data on health and health care disparities.
2. Foundations and endowments with an emphasis on cultural competence.
3. Educational modules, self-assessments, cultural competence curricula
4. Health care interpreting and translation.
5. Complementary and alternative medicine.
6. Information about specific cultural groups (ethnicity, country, religion, sexual orientation).
7. Additional resources/sites that have useful information in relation to specific issues.

Health Disparities and Diversity
Agency for Health Care Quality and Research: http://www.ahrq.gov/qual/measurix.htm
The Agency for Health Care Quality and Research of the US Department of Health and Human Services supports improvements in health outcomes; supports efforts to improve patient safety and reduce medical error; identifies strategies to improve health care access, foster appropriate use, and reduce unnecessary expenditures. On its website, you will find the annual National Healthcare Disparities Reports (NHDR). *'The NHDR is complemented by its companion report, the National Healthcare Quality Report (NHQR), which uses the same quality measures as the NHDR to provide a comprehensive overview of the quality of health care in America. Both reports measure health care quality and track changes over time but with different orientations. The NHQR addresses the current state of health care quality and the opportunities for improvement for all Americans as a whole. This perspective is useful for identifying where we are doing well as a Nation and where more work is needed. The NHDR addresses the distribution of improvements in health care quality and access across the different populations that make up America.'*

California Center for Health Statistics: http://www.dhs.ca.gov/hisp/chs/OHIR/reports/
The California Center for Health Statistics Office of Information and Research provides a wide variety of data reports related to the health status of Californians. Of particular interest are the annual County Health Status Profiles that provide comparative data for all California counties in relation to each other and to the *Healthy People 2010* goals. Other data include deaths by zip code, and statistics for many disease states and causes of death.

Center for Health Equality at the Drexel School of Public Health: http://publichealth.drexel.edu/che/
This website describes publications, resources and projects dedicated to health equity and the eradication of health disparities, particularly in urban settings. *'Drexel University's Center for Health Equality (CHE) was established to serve as major resource for addressing inequities in health and health care. By developing new information and strategies, and creating constructive partnerships with communities, government, health care providers and other academic centers, CHE will work to improve the health and well-being of the city, the state, and the nation. Its related activities will focus on three major areas: health disparities, cultural competence and health literacy.'*

Disparities Solutions Center at Massachusetts General Hospital: http://www.massgeneral.org/disparitiessolutions/index.html
Extensive and useful resources and guides are available at this policy and clinical website. *'The DSC is dedicated to the development and implementation of strategies that advance policy and practice to eliminate racial and ethnic disparities in health care. Our goal is to move beyond research and begin to take action – by developing and disseminating models for identifying and addressing racial and ethnic disparities in health care nationally, regionally, and locally. Through our work, we hope to move all health care stakeholders one step forward – and closer to eliminating racial/ethnic disparities in health care.'*

Diversity in the Health Care Workforce: http://www.nap.edu/books/030909125X/html/
This report was produced by the Institute of Medicine, and is entitled: *In the Nation's Compelling Interest: Ensuring Diversity in the Health Care Workforce* (2004). The abstract states that, *'the United States is rapidly becoming a more diverse nation, as demonstrated by the fact that nonwhite racial and ethnic groups will constitute a majority of the American population later in this century. The representation of many of these groups (e.g. African Americans, Hispanics, and Native Americans) within health professions, however, is far below their representation in the general population. Increasing racial and ethnic diversity among health professionals is important because evidence indicates that diversity is associated with improved access to care for racial and ethnic minority patients, greater patient choice and satisfaction, and better educational experiences for health professions students, among many other benefits.'*

Health Survey for England 2004: Health of Ethnic Minorities – Full Report: http://www. ic.nhs.uk/statistics-and-data-collections/health-and-lifestyles/health-survey-for-england/ health-survey-for-england-2004:-health-of-ethnic-minorities--full-report
This comprehensive report provides data from the 2004 Health Survey for England, providing national health disparity data for a wide array of health problems.

Healthy People 2010: http://www.healthypeople.gov/Document/tableofcontents.htm
Healthy People 2010 is managed by the United States Office of Disease Prevention and Health Promotion of the Department of Health and Human Services. It provides a large set of health objectives for the nation to achieve by the year 2010. The *Healthy People Midcourse Review* (http:// www.healthypeople.gov/data/midcourse/default.htm#pubs) assesses and reports progress toward meeting the *Healthy People 2010* goals over the first half the decade (2001–2010).

Kaiser Family Foundation – State Health Facts: http://www.statehealthfacts.org/
'Statehealthfacts.org is a project of the Henry J. Kaiser Family Foundation and is designed to provide free, up-to-date, and easy-to-use health data on all 50 states. Statehealthfacts.org provides data on more than 500 health topics and is linked to both the Kaiser Family Foundation website (www.kff.org) and KaiserNetwork.org (www.kaisernetwork.org).'

National Center for Health Statistics Annual Reports: www.cdc.gov/nchs/data/hus/hus06. pdf
Health, United States 2006, with Chartbook on Trends in the Health of Americans provides data for the US in comparison to other nations and a wide variety of health data and comparisons including those by race, ethnicity, gender and age. Downloads as a PDF document.

National Women's Law Center: Making the Grade on Women's Health: A National and State-by-State Report Card: http://www.nwlc.org/details.cfm?id=1861&section=health
This site provides the *2004 Report Card* with data for each state, as well as fact sheets for specific areas including: Low-Income Women's Access to Care, Access to Specific Services, The Health of Teenagers, The Health of Older and Midlife Women, and Racial and Ethnic Disparities in Healthcare. The *2004 Report Card* was the third in a series assessing the overall health of women at national and state levels. The *Report Card* was designed to promote the health and well-being of women in the US by providing a comprehensive assessment of women's health. It includes 34 health status indicators and 67 health policy indicators and provides data on progress in relation to each. The *Report Card* also provides an important overview of key disparities in the health of women based on race, ethnicity, sexual orientation, and disability status.

Public Health Agency of Canada – Reducing Health Disparities – Roles of the Health Sector: Recommended Policy Directions and Activities 2004: http://www.phac-aspc.gc.CA/ph-sp/ disparities/dr_policy_e.html
This Canadian governmental report provides statistical information on national health disparities as well as implications for policy and future directions.

Unequal Treatment (IOM Report): http://www.iom.edu/CMS/3740/4475.aspx
Access to the Institute of Medicine (IOM) Report *Unequal Treatment: Confronting Racial and Ethnic Disparities in Health Care* (2002). *'Congress, in 1999, requested an IOM study to assess the extent of disparities in the types and quality of health services received by US racial and ethnic minorities and*

non-minorities; explore factors that may contribute to inequities in care; and recommend policies and practices to eliminate these inequities. The report from that study, Unequal Treatment: Confronting Racial and Ethnic Disparities in Health Care, found that a consistent body of research demonstrates significant variation in the rates of medical procedures by race, even when insurance status, income, age, and severity of conditions are comparable. This research indicates that US racial and ethnic minorities are less likely to receive even routine medical procedures and experience a lower quality of health services.'

Foundations and Endowments with Emphasis on Cultural Competence

The California Endowment: http://www.calendow.org/
The California Endowment plays a critical and central role in improving health and health care and eliminating health disparities. The Publications and Resources section on the website offers an impressive array of curricula, data, and resources, arranged in categories such as 'Cultural Competence', 'Disparities in Health', and 'Multicultural Health Matters'.

Commonwealth Fund: http://www.cmwf.org/
This website contains various studies on health disparities from The Commonwealth Fund. *'The Commonwealth Fund is a private foundation that aims to promote a high performing health care system that achieves better access, improved quality, and greater efficiency, particularly for society's most vulnerable, including low-income people, the uninsured, minority Americans, young children, and elderly adults. The Fund carries out this mandate by supporting independent research on health care issues and making grants to improve health care practice and policy.'*

Educational Modules, Self-Assessments, Cultural Competence Curricula

Association of American Medical Colleges (AAMC) Tool for Assessment of Cultural Competence Training (TACCT): http://www.aamc.org/meded/tacct/start.htm
This site includes AAMC resources in relation to teaching cultural competence, including the TACCT, a resource guide, bibliography, and a brochure that describes the background and context for the TACCT initiative, *Cultural Competence Education for Medical Students: Assessing and Revising Curriculum.*

Centers for Disease Control Office of Minority Health and Health Disparities: http://www. cdc.gov/omhd/About/about.htm
Obtain data on health disparities at the Center for Disease Control. This website contains reports and publications on minority health resources as well as racial and ethnic minority populations. The website provides this Guiding Principle for Improving Minority Health: *'The future health of the nation will be determined to a large extent by how effectively we work with communities to reduce and eliminate health disparities between non-minority and minority populations experiencing disproportionate burdens of disease, disability, and premature death.'*

Cultural Competence Resources for Health Care Providers: http://www.hrsa.gov/ culturalcompetence/curriculumguide/
This website, provided under the auspices of the US Department of Health and Human Services, Health Resources and Services Administration is a veritable treasure chest of curricula, support materials, and resources. It is thorough, comprehensive, and creative, and can be used to guide and supplement the development and implementation of a cultural medicine curriculum.

Cultural Competency Curriculum Modules (CCCM): http://www.thinkculturalhealth.org/
The Cultural Competency Curriculum Modules (CCCM) from the Office of Minority Health, *'are grounded on the principles outlined in the* National Standards for Culturally and Linguistically Appropriate Services (CLAS) in Health Care *issued in December 2000 and serve as a first step in providing training in cultural competence to health care providers.'* This nine-hour training is divided into three overall themes: 1. Culturally Competent Care; 2. Language Access Services; and 3. Organizational Supports; and provides a thorough overview of the CLAS Standards. Furthermore, the training elements are built around clinical cases that highlight cultural and linguistic clinical and organizational dilemmas and challenges. The program is creative and engaging, with brief videos of the introductory cases. It offers interactive opportunities for reflecting on the material presented, as well as numerous links for further reading and exploration of themes of interest. This interactive program provides nine continuing medical

education units to those who complete the entire curriculum. Although it is aimed toward family physicians, it is appropriate for all health professions students.

DHHS Office of Minority Health Resource Center: http://www.omhrc.gov/
This website contains the US Department of Health and Human Services (DHHS) Office of Minority Health Resource Center. *'The mission of the Office of Minority Health (OMH) is to improve and protect the health of racial and ethnic minority populations through the development of health policies and programs that will eliminate health disparities.'* These include public health programs affecting American Indians and Alaska Natives, Asian Americans, Blacks/African-Americans, Hispanics/Latinos, Native Hawaiians, and other Pacific Islanders. This site has information in three categories: staying healthy, health disparities, and communities in action. Within the health disparities area is a link to the web-based training CME program: *A Physicians Practical Guide to Cultural Competence*. The site also includes discussions on a variety of health topics.

Diversity Rx: http://www.diversityrx.org/
This site has a variety of resources linked to it. It includes a multicultural health best practices overview that covers: 1. culturally competent health services; 2. policy development and research in multicultural health; and 3. community capacity building. Within the overview, links are provided to cultural competence training programs throughout the US. The site also provides links to interpreter services and guidelines for practice as well as an active and informative listserv. Diversity Rx is supported by: The National Conference of State Legislatures (NCSL), Resources for Cross Cultural Health Care (RCCHC), The Henry J. Kaiser Family Foundation of Menlo Park, CA. Editor: Julia Puebla Fortier.

Maternal and Child Health (MCH) Library: http://mchlibrary.info/KnowledgePaths/kp_race.html
'This knowledge path has been compiled by the Maternal and Child Health (MCH) Library at Georgetown University. It presents a selection of current, high-quality resources about identifying and eliminating racial and ethnic disparities in health. The path is aimed at health professionals, program administrators, policymakers, researchers, and families, and it will be updated periodically.'

Medscape Health Diversity Resource Center: http://www.medscape.com
This website offers a rich array of clinically applicable health diversity and health disparity information. Content is offered in the areas of sex and gender, race/ethnicity, religion and culture, socioeconomic status, and physical/mental disability. Recent journal articles are summarized in the 'news' section, and the site offers a number of opportunities for continuing medical education in these arenas.

National Center for Cultural Competence (NCCC): http://www11.georgetown.edu/research/gucchd/nccc/
'The mission of the National Center for Cultural Competence (NCCC) is to increase the capacity of health and mental health programs to design, implement, and evaluate culturally and linguistically competent service delivery systems.' This site includes a self-assessment instrument, the Health Practitioner Cultural Competence Assessment, comprised of six subscales: values and belief systems, cultural aspects of epidemiology, clinical decision-making, life cycle events, cross-cultural communication, and empowerment/health management.

PBS Frontline, A Class Divided: http://www.pbs.org/wgbh/pages/frontline/shows/divided/
The website for 'A Class Divided' describes the *'encore presentation of the classic documentary on third-grade teacher Jane Elliott's 'blue eyes/brown eyes' exercise, originally conducted in the days following the assassination of Reverend Martin Luther King Jr. in 1968'*. This website describes the *'daring lesson on discrimination'* and is *'designed to help you use the film to engage (participants) in reflection and dialogue about the historical role of racism in the United States, as well as the role of prejudice and stereotyping in (participants') lives today'*. This page contains links for the PBS show Frontline report on the original classroom exercise done by Jane Elliot.

PBS Race Website: http://www.pbs.org/race
Race: The Power of an Illusion is the online companion to the California Newsreel's three-part documentary about race in society, science, and history. A statement from the series Executive

Producer and Co-Director of California Newsreel, Larry Adelman, explains the basis for the documentary and this accompanying website, *'What is this thing called "race?" – a question so basic it is rarely raised. What we discovered is that most of our common assumptions about race – for instance, that the world's people can be divided biologically along racial lines – are wrong. Yet the consequences of racism are very real. How do we make sense of these two seeming contradictions? Our hope is that this series can help us all navigate through our myths and misconceptions, and scrutinize some of the assumptions we take for granted. In that sense, the real subject of the film (and website) is not so much race but the viewer, or more precisely, the notions about race we all hold.'*

PBS – What is Race Page: http://www.pbs.org/race/001_WhatIsRace/001_00-home.htm
This page of the PBS Race website titled 'What is Race' gives users ten facts about race. These 10 facts are answers to many of the misconceptions about race.

PBS – Sorting People Page: http://www.pbs.org/race/002_SortingPeople/002_00-home.htm
This page of the PBS Race website asks the questions, *'How easy is it to group people into "races" based on appearance? What about using individual traits? Does everybody classify the same way? Try your hand at "sorting" individuals and see if it matches how people think of themselves. Or explore how we might sort people by physical traits.'* On this site you will see pictures of individuals and have to match them with the current racial categories of the US Census. Once this is done, you can click to see how many you correctly classified, and find out how they classify themselves.

PBS – Where Race Lives Page: http://www.pbs.org/race/006_WhereRaceLives/006_00home.htm
On the PBS Race website, the page 'Where Race Lives' has several exercises to explore. *The site asks, 'Where you live in the US isn't just a matter of preference. It's also about providing for the future. Does everyone have the same access to home ownership, good schools, and resources? Explore how government policies and past discrimination have made generating wealth easier for some Americans than others'.* By clicking on 'A Tale of Two Families' you will explore this issue by looking at two individuals and how their 'race' affected their family wealth.

On this page, you can also click on 'The Downward Spiral' which asks the questions *'How does a good neighborhood "turn bad"? What triggers the decline of an area? Some people claim that once minorities move in, the neighborhood starts to deteriorate. There is a chain of events that will cause even the most affluent area to become an impoverished one. But it's not about who's moving in – it's about who leaves.'* This page shows how 'White Flight' can cause a downward spiral in a neighborhood.

Project Implicit and the Implicit Association Test (IAT): https://implicit.harvard.edu/implicit/
Project Implicit is the name of a Harvard University research project that has been combined with educational outreach in their 'virtual laboratory' the IAT website, where your learners can examine their own hidden biases. The IAT has been available on this website since 1998. On the site you can also find results to date from the over 4.5 million demonstration tests that have been taken. The IATs available on the site include: Race IAT, Arab-Muslim IAT, Gender-Science IAT, Weapons-Race IAT, President IAT, Age IAT, Native American-White IAT, Judaism-Other Religions IAT, Disabled-Abled IAT, Gender-Career IAT, Gay-Straight IAT, Asian-European American IAT. As there are so many choices, learners should be directed to complete one or two that relate specifically to the objectives of your session or curriculum.

Physicians for Human Rights: http://physiciansforhumanrights.org/
The site includes descriptions of many projects including an *'annotated bibliography of key articles in the peer-reviewed literature on racial and ethnic disparities in medical care (http://phr-equaltreatment. org/). These have been organized into 17 disease or clinical categories; four additional sections present the related but non-categorical issues of clinical trials, research methods, patient trust, and cultural competency.'*

Provider's Guide to Quality and Culture: http://erc.msh.org/mainpage.cfm?file=1.0.htm&module=provider&language=English
The Manager's Electronic Resource Center contains The Provider's Guide to Quality and Culture. *'This website is designed to assist health care organizations throughout the US in providing*

high quality, culturally competent services to multi-ethnic populations.' The Provider's Guide to Quality and Culture is a joint project of Management Sciences for Health (MSH), US Department of Health and Human Services, Health Resources and Services Administration, Bureau of Primary Health Care. The Provider's Guide has information in a wide variety of areas including patient–provider interaction (e.g. clinical exchanges, prior assumptions and prejudices; medical history and diagnosis, patient adherence); health disparities (with links to key data sources); cultural groups and culturally competent organizations.

Race, Health Care and the Law: http://academic.udayton.edu/health/index.htm
'The Race, Health Care and the Law website of the University of Dayton is dedicated to improving the health status of persons who are discriminated against based on race and/or ethnicity (with specific attention on African Americans, Asian Americans, Latino (a) Americans, Native Americans, and Pacific Americans). We approach this goal by helping legislators, policy makers, lawyers, health care professionals and consumers examine race, health, and human rights, with particular attention on the role of domestic and international law in promoting and/or eliminating racial disparities in health status and health care.'

Tolerance.org (Southern Poverty Law Center): http://www.tolerance.org/index.jsp
This website provides a Hidden Bias Primer and is linked to the Project Implicit and the Implicit Association Test (IAT) website. It includes a description of hidden bias and definitions of terms like stereotype and discrimination, as well as sections entitled 'About Stereotypes and Prejudices', 'The Effects of Bias and Stereotypes' and 'What Can You Do About Unconscious Stereotypes and Prejudices?' This last section can assist health professions instructors in debriefing sessions on bias and stereotyping as it provides concrete steps to address issues that the learners may have been unaware of or unwilling to admit prior to the cultural competence session. The site also provides a variety of resources including '101 Tools for Tolerance' and '10 Ways to Fight Hate on Campus'.

Understanding Prejudice (Social Psychology Network): http://www.understandingprejudice.org.
This is *'A website for students, teachers, and others interested in the causes and consequences of prejudice.'* This site contains prejudice resources such as searchable databases, exercises and demonstrations, multimedia center, and a teacher's corner with information to assist college instructors, although these tips can also assist teachers of health care professionals. It includes a pretest that the learners can access at a later date to review. If the learners enter a prearranged 'course code' the teacher can access the writings of the students. The site could be used in a pre-post assessment of attitudes and knowledge in relation to prejudice.

Unnatural Causes: www.unnaturalcauses.org
This is the website companion to the documentary series by the same name shown on PBS. Both the documentary and the website powerfully explore racial and socioeconomic inequalities in health. The website includes video clips from the documentary as well as discussion guides. Furthermore, one can explore case examples, which put a human face on health disparities, and there are seven 'learn-by-doing' experiential exercises. Finally, the resources section offers a treasure of online health equity resources.

Health Care Interpreting and Translation

California Healthcare Interpreting Association: http://chiaonline.org/content/view/42/100/
'California Healthcare Interpreting Association (CHIA) is a 501 (c) (3) public charity dedicated to improving the quality and availability of language services in the delivery of health care. The organization was founded as the California Healthcare Interpreters Association in 1996 by a group of interpreters and program managers. The name was changed in 2003 to "Interpreting" to better reflect CHIA's mission of serving the public interest, and particularly the interests of (Limited English Proficient) LEP patients, rather than serving as a professional association of interpreters.'

Cross Cultural Care Program (Seattle): http://www.xculture.org/
'Through a combination of cultural competency trainings, interpreter trainings, research projects, community coalition building, and other services, the (Cross-Cultural Health Care Program) CCHCP serves as a bridge between communities and health care institutions to ensure full access to quality

health care that is culturally and linguistically appropriate.' This website contains information on books, videos, and articles relevant to health care interpreting. It has extensive information on immigrant communities in Seattle and provides a model of these types of descriptions.

Free2Professional Translation: http://www.freetranslation.com/free/
'Free2Professional Translation is wholly owned by SDL International, a leading globalization company. SDL'e Enterprise Translation Server is the most powerful automatic translation engine on the market today and powers Free2Professional Translation's instant translation service. Free2Professional Translation allows users to obtain free translations of both text and web pages. The translation is generated by a computer, displayed instantly, and the user is dynamically shown the cost of having the same text professionally translated or edited by Click2Translate Express.' Caution: care should be taken whenever using a computer-generated translation service as they may not provide the most accurate material.

University of California, Los Angeles Language Materials Project: http://www.lmp.ucla.edu/
'The UCLA Language Materials Project (LMP) is an online bibliographic database of teaching and learning materials for over 100 Less Commonly Taught Languages (LCTLs). Full bibliographic information is provided for each item in the database, including detailed annotations that describe the content and other features of the material, intended to help you find the most appropriate materials to meet your individual teaching and learning needs. When possible, we provide information on how to order materials. The LMP does not sell the materials found on the database.'

Complementary and Alternative Medicine
National Center for Complementary and Alternative Medicine (NCCAM): http://nccam.nih.gov/
NCCAM is part of the National Institutes of Health and is *'dedicated to exploring complementary and alternative healing practices in the context of rigorous science, training complementary and alternative medicine (CAM) researchers, and disseminating authoritative information to the public and professionals.'* It supports clinical and basic science research projects in CAM by awarding grants as well as conducting its own studies. It also awards grants that provide training and career development opportunities for researchers. In addition, NCCAM studies ways to integrate evidence-based CAM practices into conventional medical practice, and supports programs to develop models for incorporating CAM into the curriculum of medical, dental, and nursing schools.

Natural Medicine's Comprehensive Database: http://www.naturaldatabase.com/
'The database provides all of the clinically relevant information in an easy-to-use format.' The database allows product searching from any page. Patient handouts for each product are found on the site, along with lists of references with their abstracts. The site includes effectiveness ratings on projects which are updated as new scientific evidence is reported. This database states that it *'provides the most comprehensive listing of brand name product ingredients available.'*

Information about Specific Cultural Groups
A wide variety of health care and educational institutions have websites that provide information about various cultures, religions, and other minority groups. Below are a selected few provided in alphabetical order by web address: http://bearspace.baylor.edu/Charles_Kemp/www/refugees.htm

This site provides resources for cross-cultural care and prevention in relation to a variety of Asian cultures including Burmese, Cambodian/Khmer, Laotian/Lao, Vietnamese, Indian (Asian), as well as information on the refugees and immigrant health.

http://www.beliefnet.com/index/index_10000.html
This site provides useful, neutrally written descriptions of 28 different faiths and their belief structures including Buddhism, Hinduism, Christianity (many variants), Islam, Judaism, Pagan and earth-based Taoism, and Sikhism.

http://www.ethnomed.org/
This website contains culture-specific pages as well as pages on cross-cultural health topics. The site is maintained by the University of Washington. When visited in January 2007 the site had

cultural profiles for the following cultural groups: Cambodian, Chinese, Eritrean, Ethiopian (also Oromo and Tigrean people), Hmong, Mexican, Somali, and Vietnamese.

http://www.health.qld.gov.au/multicultural/health_workers/cultdiver_guide.asp
This Queensland, Australia site provides health care information about a number of cultural groups including Bosnian Muslims, Cambodians, Chinese, Croatians, Greeks, Hmong, Italians, Muslims from West Asia, Philippines, Samoans, Tongans, Serbians, and Vietnamese.

http://www.healthsystem.virginia.edu/internet/chaplaincy/
This site provides a booklet entitled *Religious Beliefs and Practices Affecting Health Care* developed for use by UVA Health System staff. Hard copies of the booklet are available for $3/copy or $30/ dozen. The PDF file is also available for $25 and allows the purchaser to make and distribute copies at their own institution.

http://www.hispanichealth.org/
This site has resources for purchase including: *Delivering Health Care to Hispanics: A Manual for Providers* 3rd edition (2004) and the (2004) Companion Workbook; and *A Primer for Cultural Proficiency: Towards Quality Health Services for Hispanics* (2001).

http://www.metrokc.gov/health/glbt/
These webpages address the health concerns of gay, lesbian, bisexual, and transgender people, also known as 'GLBT' people and 'sexual minorities'.

http://www.msmc.la.edu/ccf/LAC.Korean.html
This site has a very useful description of the Korean-American community in Los Angeles.

Additional Resources
Anti-Defamation League: http://www.adl.org/
The Anti-Defamation League Charter reads, *'The immediate object of the League is to stop, by appeals to reason and conscience and, if necessary, by appeals to law, the defamation of the Jewish people. Its ultimate purpose is to secure justice and fair treatment to all citizens alike and to put an end forever to unjust and unfair discrimination against, and ridicule of, any sect or body of citizens.'* Although the primarily focus of this organization and its website is on anti-Semitism, it also has articles and resources on 'hate' in general and the corresponding issue of civil rights.

Bafá Bafá: http://www.stsintl.com/
The Simulation Training Systems website offers Bafá Bafá for purchase. This is a wonderfully engaging experiential simulation game that facilitates learning about cultural and linguistic differences. Fun to play, and rich with intercultural learning, the materials for this simulation game are available for purchase on the website. Bafá Bafá would be a great addition to a retreat or longer training workshop on cultural aspects of health.

Barnga (Intercultural Press): http://www.interculturalpress.com
Barnga is a very entertaining interactive learning game that facilitates experiential learning about cross-cultural communication, rule navigation and social mobility. All necessary materials and debriefing guide are available for purchase on the website. This would work especially well on a retreat or for a longer training workshop. Other intriguing and helpful resources are also available through Intercultural Press on topics such as Dispute Resolution and Conflict, Diversity, Health, Intercultural Education and Training, Latino Culture and Understanding Culture.

California Newsreel: http://www.newsreel.org/nav/topics.asp?cat=3
The California Newsreel's section on Diversity Training and Multiculturalism has 29 films available for purchase including the famous films related to the blue-eye, brown-eye training and the films of the PBS series, *Race – The Power of an Illusion*. All of the videos in this collection could be used as tools in diversity training and discussions. However, these tend to be longer videos (30 minutes to one hour) that would require previewing and making careful selections of segment for directed teaching.

Educational Consultants: www.galindoconsultants.com
Educational Consultants, Inc. offers services to churches and educational institutions. Its Resources section provides links to a variety of books and other resources including one used in this curriculum: Galindo I, Boomer E, Reagan D. *A Family Genogram Workbook*. Nebraska: Educational Consultants, Inc.; 2006.

Fanlight Productions: http://www.fanlight.com/home.php
Fanlight Productions distributes film and video on the social issues in a variety of areas including: health care, mental health, professional ethics, aging and gerontology, disabilities, gender, and sexuality. They distribute the *Worlds Apart* videos as well as a variety of other video resources that might be used in cultural competence training.

Museum of Tolerance: http://www.museumoftolerance.com/
The Museum of Tolerance (Los Angeles) website contains a Teacher's Guide as well as an Online Learning and Resources section. The site contains the following description of the museum: '*The Museum of Tolerance is a high tech, hands-on experiential museum that focuses on two central themes through unique interactive exhibits: the dynamics of racism and prejudice in America and the history of the Holocaust – the ultimate example of man's inhumanity to man. The Museum, the educational arm of the Simon Wiesenthal Center, was founded to challenge visitors to confront bigotry and racism, and to understand the Holocaust in both historic and contemporary contexts. The genesis of the Museum, the first of its kind in the world, came from the leadership of the Simon Wiesenthal Center, the internationally recognized Jewish human rights organization named in honor of Simon Wiesenthal.*'

National Multi-Cultural Institute: http://www.nmci.org/
'*Founded in 1983, the National Multi-Cultural Institute (NMCI) is proud to be one of the first organizations to have recognized the nation's need for new services, knowledge, and skills in the growing field of multiculturalism and diversity. NMCI's mission is to work with individuals, organizations, and communities in creating a society that is strengthened and empowered by its diversity. Through its initiatives, NMCI leads efforts to increase communication, understanding and respect among people of diverse backgrounds and addresses some of the important systemic issues of multiculturalism facing our society. This is accomplished through conferences in the Spring and Fall, individualized organizational training and consulting interventions, publications, and leading edge projects.*'

New York Times Company, About Race Relations: http://racerelations.about.com/
The About Race Relations website contains current events, definitions of key terms and concepts, as well as a variety of articles addressing the intersection of race and other relevant social issues or groups. The emphasis on this site is recent stories in the news and links to legal rights.

WordPress, The White Privilege Website: http://www.whiteprivilege.com/
The White Privilege website is a free resource for antiracism education and activism; its editorial focus is analyzing and critically assessing social privilege based on race. It contains articles, essays, and poetry related to the subject of white privilege. The term is defined and many links to other relevant sites are provided. This is an excellent site to find literary pieces that you can use in narrative assignments.

Video/DVD Resources

America in Black and White: Healthcare the Great Divide. ABC News Productions, 1999 Feb 24 (23 minutes).

> Focus: health care disparities.
> Level: awareness, some knowledge (dated).
> Overview: the portion on physician responsibility in relation to disparities is very good – could help increase awareness of unintentional bias. Suggested clip: the approximately 14 minutes from the introduction by Ted Koppel of 'today's topic' to the statement that next he will talk with the Surgeon General. There is one 'station break' in the middle of this section that could serve as a pause point for discussion.

The Angry Heart. Fanlight Productions, 2001 (57 minutes).
http://www.fanlight.com/catalog/films/331_ah.php

> Focus: racial/ethnic health disparities.
> Level: awareness, some knowledge (dated).
> Overview: this is a documentary video account of an African-American man with cardiac disease. The video highlights racial disparities in disease as well as the role of culture, family and spirituality in the healing process. The documentary includes commentary from leading researchers in the field of racial health disparities.

Communicating Effectively Through an Interpreter. Cross Cultural Health Care Program, Seattle Washington, 1998 (28 minutes).
http://www.xculture.org/NWRC_Catalog.php

> Focus: use of an interpreter (trained or untrained).
> Level: skill development.
> Overview: this tape effectively guides the teaching of the correct use of an interpreter.

Cultural Issues in the Clinical Setting Series A and B. Kaiser Permanente, 2002 (70 minutes). To order call: (323) 259–4546.

> Focus: a variety of cultural issues.
> Level: cultural awareness for all 'clips' with the *Sickle Cell in the ER* both short and powerful; some knowledge in the gay teenager with an STD, the lesbian pregnancy and the Hmong birth; positive demonstration of skill in the gay teenager scene and in the side conversation within the Hmong segment.
> Overview: wide variety of topics as described below with many a good length for triggering discussion.

Series A:
1. *Diabetic Compliance* (Latino). Language barriers, unskilled interpreter. Scene A: negative example (7:15 minutes), Scene B: positive example (9:14 minutes).
2. *Sickle Cell in the ER* (4:43 minutes). Young African-American male, unrecognized bias, patient did not receive needed care.
3. *Pediatric Asthma* (7:09 minutes). Provider and family from different cultures (communication issues).
4. *A Somatic Complaint* (6:07 minutes). Provider (white male) and patient (Asian female) – communication issues.
5. *Prostate Exam* (3:55 minutes). African-American patient and physician, fear of the prostate exam, man ran out and did not have the needed exam.
6. *Gay Adolescent* (11:19 minutes). STD, confidentiality. Positive example of an interview with a young gay teen who is sexually active.

Series B:
Beyond Obstetrics: Birthing Issues – Four Cultural Perspectives (18:20 minutes).
1. Lesbian pregnancy: not typical pregnancy.
2. Hmong: a jacket for the soul.
3. Latino: a big baby is coming.
4. Somalia: female circumcision and c-section.

Eye of the Storm and later videos of Jane Elliott's work on power and discrimination. Trainer's Toolchest. Search details and ordering information at http://www.trainerstoolchest.com

First Do No Harm. Partnership for Patient Safety, 2001.
http://www.p4ps.org/interactive_videos.asp
 Focus: patient-center, system-based approach to patient safety.
 Level: awareness, attitudes, knowledge.
 Overview: an interactive video series with an accompanying facilitator's guide.
  Part 1: *A Case Study of Systems Failure* (18 minutes drama, 50 minutes optional discussion).
  Part 2: *Taking the Lead* (19 minutes drama, 35 minutes discussion). Reaction to an adverse event.
  Part 3: *Healing Lives, Changing Cultures* (26 minutes drama, 61 minutes discussion). Resolves the issues raised in parts 1 and 2.

Quality Care for Diverse Populations. American Academy of Family Physicians, 2002 (50 minutes).
http://www.aafp.org/online/en/home/cme/selfstudy/qualitycarevideo.html
 Focus: variety of cross-cultural issues.
 Level: skill development.
 Overview: this is an entire curriculum complete with a notebook of materials with short vignettes that can be used to teach the AAFP mnemonics.
 1. Pregnant Hispanic women, little English, use of interpreter, introduces mnemonic BATHE (Background, Affect [how it is affecting you], Trouble [what is troubling you], Handling [how are you Handling things that trouble you], Empathy).
 2. Obesity, adolescence and diabetes, African-American overweight male, introduces mnemonic LEARN (Listen, Explain, Acknowledge, Recommend, Negotiate) for identifying cultural identity factors.
 3. Sexual orientation, African-American woman, lesbian, dealing with families on their own terms.
 4. Immigrant health care, Vietnamese immigrant, cross-cultural health care, introduces ETHNIC (Explanation, Treatment, Healers (traditional), Negotiate, Intervention, Collaboration).
 5. Cross-cultural end-of-life issues with a Native American elderly couple.

Unnatural Causes. Vital Pictures and California Newsreel, 2008 (4 hours).
www.unnaturalcauses.org
 Focus: an outstanding seven-part (four-hour) documentary on racial and economic inequality in health disparities.
 Level: cultural awareness and knowledge.
 Overview: the series explores connections between health and skin color, infant mortality health disparities, the 'Latino Paradox' in which new immigrants are healthier than seasoned immigrants, diabetes prevalence in American Indian communities, TB rates, impacts of job loss on health, and the contributors of geography (where one lives) to health status.

Worlds Apart. Fanlight Productions, 2003 (four videos).
http://www.fanlight.com/catalog/films/331_ah.php
 Focus: each tape has a different focus, described below.
 Level: cultural awareness.
 Overview: these are a bit long for a video clip if shown in total. They raise issues that require skilled facilitation in learner discussion to move learner attitudes and result in individual increase in desire for more knowledge or skills.
 1. *Mohammed Kochi's Story* (14:05 minutes). This vignette focuses on how culture (including religious beliefs) influences the way families make medical decisions, how acculturation can affect health beliefs, and the importance of using an interpreter with Limited English Proficient (LEP) patients.
 2. *Justine Chitsena's Story* (11:19 minutes). In this vignette, the focus is on how culture influences health beliefs (explanatory models), the use of Complementary and Alternative Medicine (CAM), as well as barriers and tools to effective cross-cultural communication.

3. *Robert Phillips' Story* (10:08 minutes). The video promotes discussion of discrimination and health disparities, provider stereotyping, and patient mistrust of the medical community.
4. *Alicia Mercado's Story* (12:56 minutes). This vignette stresses the importance of patient's perspective on chronic disease, social stressors, and cultural factors which can influence non-adherence to treatment recommendations.

Reference Books

Adams M, Blumenfeld WJ, Castaneda R, *et al. Readings for Diversity and Social Justice: An Anthology on Racism, Sexism, Anti-semitism, Heterosexism, Classism and Ableism.* New York: Routledge; 2000.

Alexander M, Lenahan P, Pavlov A, editors. *Cinemeducation: A Comprehensive Guide to Using Film in Medical Education.* Oxford, UK: Radcliffe Publishing; 2005.

Anderson JB. *Speaking to Groups: Eyeball to eyeball.* Vienna, VA: Windmoor Press; 1989.

Anderson NB, Bulatao RA, Cohen B, editors. *Critical Perspectives On Racial And Ethnic Differences In Health In Late Life.* Washington, DC: National Academies Press; 2004.

Bigby J, editor. *Cross Cultural Medicine.* Philadelphia: American College of Physicians –American Society of Internal Medicine; 2003.

Byrd WM, Clayton L. *An American Health Dilemma: A medical history of African Americans and the problem of race: Beginnings to 1900.* New York: Routledge; 2000.

Byrd WM. Clayton L. *An American Health Dilemma: Race, medicine and health care in the United States 1900 –2000.* New York: Routledge; 2002.

Campinha-Bacote J. *The Process of Cultural Competence in the Delivery of Health Care Services: A culturally competent model of care.* 3rd ed. Cincinnati, OH: Transcultural CARE Associates; 1999.

Campo R. *What the Body Told.* Durham, NC: Duke University Press; 1996. pp. 70.

Culhane-Pera K, Vawter DE, Xiong P, *et al.*, editors. *Healing by Heart: Clinical and Ethical Case Stories of Hmong Families and Western Providers.* Nashville, TN: Vanderbilt University Press; 2003.

Demons JL, Celez R. Geriatrics and end-of-life care. In: Satcher D, Pamies R, editors. *Multicultural Medicine and Health Disparities.* New York: McGraw Hill; 2006.

Fadiman A. *The Spirit Catches You and You Fall Down.* New York: Farrar, Straus, Giroux; 1998.

Fisher R, Ury W. *Getting to Yes: Negotiation agreement without giving in.* New York: Penguin Books; 1983.

Gladwell M. *Blink: The power of thinking without thinking.* New York: Little Brown and Company; 2005.

Gregory K, Peck MG, Davidson EC. Pregnancy and women's health. In: Satcher D, Pamies R, editors. *Multicultural Medicine and Health Disparities.* New York: McGraw-Hill; 2006. pp. 105–26.

Hummer RA, Benjamins MR, Rogers RG. *Racial and Ethnic Disparities in Health and Mortality Among the U.S. Elderly Population.* Washington, DC: National Academies Press; 2004.

Kaiser Permanente. *A Providers Handbook on Culturally Competent Care: African American population.* Oakland: Kaiser; 2000.

Kaiser Permanente. *A Providers Handbook on Culturally Competent Care: Asian and Pacific Island American populations.* Oakland: Kaiser; 2000.

Kaiser Permanente. *A Providers Handbook on Culturally Competent Care: Latino population.* Oakland: Kaiser; 2000.

Kaiser Permanente. *A Providers Handbook on Culturally Competent Care: Lesbian, gay, bisexual and transgendered population.* Oakland: Kaiser; 2000.

Kawachi I, Kennedy B, Wilkinson R, editors. *The Society and Population Health Reader: Income inequality and health.* New York: The New Press; 1999.

Kleinman A. *The Illness Narratives: Suffering, healing, and the human condition,* New York: Basic Books; 1988.

Kohn, LT, Corrigan, JM and Donaldson, MS. *To Err is Human: Building a Safer Health System.* (IOM Report). Washington DC: National Academies Press; 2000.

Krieger N, editor. *Embodying Inequality: Epidemiologic perspectives.* Amityville, NY: Baywood Publishing; 2005.

LaVeist T, editor. *A Public Health Reader: Race, ethnicity and health.* San Francisco: Jossey-Bass; 2002.

Lu FG, Lim R, Mezzich JE. Issues in the assessment and diagnosis of culturally diverse individuals. In: Oldham J, Riba M, editors. *Review of Psychiatry.* Vol. 14. Washington DC: American Psychiatric Press; 1995. pp. 477–510.

Meyer I, Northridge M. *The Health of Sexual Minorities: Public health perspectives on lesbian, gay, bisexual and transgender populations.* New York: Springer Publications; 2006.

Minkler M, editor. *Community organizing and community building for health.* New Jersey: The Rutgers State University; 1999.

National Standards for Culturally and Linguistically Appropriate Services in Health Care: Final report. Rockville, MD: US Department of Health and Human Services, Office of Minority Health; 2001 Mar.

Pinderhughes E. *Understanding Race, Ethnicity and Power.* New York: The Free Press; 1989.

Rhyne R, Bogue R, Kukulka G, *et al.*, editors. *Community-Oriented Primary Care: Health care for the 21st century.* Washington DC: American Public Health Association; 1998.

Salimbene S. *CLAS A–Z: A practical guide for implementing the National Standards for Culturally and Linguistically Appropriate Services (CLAS) in health care.* Rockford, IL: Inter-Face Intl.; 2002. Available from: http://www.omhrc.gov/templates/browse.aspx?lvl=1&lvlID=13

Satcher D, Pamies R. *Multicultural Medicine and Health Disparities.* New York: McGraw Hill; 2006.

Shankle M, editor. *The Handbook of Lesbian, Gay, Bisexual and Transgender Public Health: A practitioner's guide to service.* Binghamton, New York: Haworth Press; 2006.

Shulz A, Mullings L. *Gender, Race, Class and Health: Intersectional approaches.* San Francisco: Jossey-Bass; 2006.

Sloane P, Slatt L, Ebell M, *et al.* editors. *Essentials of Family Medicine.* Baltimore: Lippincott Williams & Wilkins; 2002.

Smedley BD, Stith AY, Nelson AR, editors. *Unequal Treatment: Confronting Racial and Ethnic Disparities in Health Care.* (IOM Report) Board on Health Sciences Policy. Washington, DC: National Academies Press; 2002. Available from: http://www.iom.edu/CMS/3740/4475.aspx

Stuart MR, Lieberman JA. *The Fifteen Minute Hour: Applied psychotherapy for the primary care physician.* 2nd ed. Westport, CT: Praeger; 1993.

Sue D. *Overcoming Our Racism: The journey to liberation.* San Francisco: Jossey-Bass; 2003.

Westberg J, Jason H. *Fostering Learning in Small Groups: A practical guide.* New York: Springer Publishing Company; 1996.

Journal Articles

Aberegg SK, Terry PB. Medical decision-making and healthcare disparities: the physician's role. *J Lab Clin Med*. 2004 Jul; **144**(1): 11–7.

Aeder L, Altshuler L, Kachur E, *et al*. The 'Culture OSCE': introducing a formative assessment into a postgraduate program. *Educ Health*. 2007 May; **20**(1): 11.

Ahmed R, Bowen J, O'Donnell W. Cultural competence and language interpreter services in Minnesota: results of a needs assessment survey administered to physician members of the Minnesota Medical Association. *Minnesota Med*. 2004 Dec; **87**(12): 40–2.

Albarran NB, Ballesteros MN, Morales GG, *et al*. Dietary behavior and type 2 diabetes care *Patient Educ Couns*. 2006 May; **61**(2): 191–9.

Alexander M, Hall MN, Pettice YJ. Cinemeducation: an innovative approach to teaching psychosocial medical care. *Fam Med*. 1994; **26**(7): 430–3.

Anderson LM, Scrimshaw SC, Fullilove MT, *et al*. Task Force on Community Preventive Services. Culturally competent healthcare systems. A systematic review. *Am J Prev Med*. 2003 Apr; **24** (3 Suppl.): 68–79.

Anderson NL, Calvillo ER, Fongwa MN. Community-based approaches to strengthen cultural competency in nursing education and practice *J Transcult Nurs*. 2007 Jan; **18**(1 Suppl.): 49S–59S; discussion 60S–67S.

Altshuler L, Kachur E. A culture OSCE: teaching residents to bridge different worlds. *Acad Med*. 2001; **76**: 514.

Assemi M, Cullander C, Hudmon KS. Psychometric analysis of a scale assessing self-efficacy for cultural competence in patient counseling. *Ann Pharmacother*. 2006 Dec; **40**(12): 2130–5.

Azer SA. Challenges facing PBL tutors: 12 tips for successful group facilitation. *Med Teach*. 2005 Dec; **27**(8): 676–81.

Bakker LJ, Cavender A. Promoting culturally competent care for gay youth. *J School Nurs*. 2003 Apr; **19**(2): 65–72.

Balsa AI, Seiler N, McGuire TG, *et al*. Clinical uncertainty and healthcare disparities. *Am J Law Med*. 2003; **29**(2–3): 203–19.

Baquet CR, Carter-Pokras O, Bengen-Seltzer B. Healthcare disparities and models for change. *Am J Manag Care*. 2004; **10**(Special Issue): SP5–SP11.

Bartol GM, Richardson L. Using Literature to Create Cultural Competence. *J Nurs Scholarsh*. 1998; **20**(1): 75–9.

Bender DE, Clawson M, Harlan C, *et al*. Improving access for Latino immigrants: evaluation of language training adapted to the needs of health professionals. *J Immigr Health*. 2004 Oct; **6**(4): 197–209.

Ber R, Alroy G. Teaching professionalism with the aid of trigger films. *Med Teach*. 2002; **24**(5): 528–31.

Ber R, Alroy G. Twenty years of experience using trigger films as a teaching tool. *Acad Med*. 2001 Jun; **76**(6): 656–8.

Bergeson SC, Dean JD. A systems approach to patient-centered care. *JAMA*. 2006 Dec 20; **296**(23): 2848–51.

Berlin FA, Fowkes WC Jr. A teaching framework for cross-cultural health care: application in family practice. *West J Med*. 1983; **139**: 934–8.

Betancourt JR. Cultural competence and medical education: many names, many perspectives, one goal. *Acad Med*. 2006 Jun; **81**(6): 499–501.

Betancourt JR, Green AR, Carrillo JE, *et al*. Defining cultural competence: a practical framework for addressing racial/ethnic disparities in health and health care. *Pub Health Rep*. 2003 Jul–Aug; **118**(4): 293–302.

Betancourt JR, Maina AW. The Institute of Medicine report 'Unequal Treatment': implications for academic health centers. *Mt Sinai J Med*. 2004 Oct; **71**(5): 314–21.

Bhui K, Warfa N, Edonya P, *et al*. Cultural competence in mental health care: a review of model evaluations. *BMC Health Serv Res*. 2007; **7**: 15.

Blake TK. Journaling; an active learning technique. *Int J Nurs Educ Scholarsh*. 2005; **2**: Article 7.

Bloche MG. Health care disparities: science, politics, and race. *N Engl J Med*. 2004 Apr 8; **350**(15): 1568–70.

Botelho R. A negotiation model for the doctor-patient relationship. *Fam Pract*. 1992; **9**(2): 210–218.

Boutin-Foster C, Foster JC, Konopasek L. Viewpoint: physician, know thyself: the professional culture of medicine as a framework for teaching cultural competence. *Acad Med*. 2008 Jan; **83**(1): 106–11.

Brathwaite AC, Majumdar B. Evaluation of a cultural competence educational programme. *J Adv Nurs*. 2006 Feb; **53**(4): 470–9.

Brazeau C, Boyd L, Crosson J. Changing an existing OSCE to a teaching tool: the making of a teaching OSCE. *Acad Med*. 2002 Sep; **77**(9): 932.

Bregman B, Irvine C. Subjectifying the Patient: creative writing and the clinical encounter. *Fam Med*. 2004; **36**(6): 400–1.

Brown SA, Blozis SA, Kouzekanani K, *et al*. Dosage effects of diabetes self-management education for Mexican Americans: the Starr County Border Health Initiative. *Diabet Care*. 2005 Mar; **28**(3): 527–32.

Browning CR, Cagney KA. Moving beyond poverty: neighborhood structure, social processes, and health. *J Health Soc Behav*. 2003 Dec; **44**(4): 552–71.

Campbell TL, McDaniel SH, Cole-Kelly K, *et al*. Family interviewing: a review of the literature in primary care. *Fam Med*. 2002 May; **34**(5): 312–8.

Carraccio C, Englander R. Evaluating competence using a portfolio: a literature review and web-based application to the ACGME competencies. *Teach Learn Med*. 2004; **16**(4): 381–7.

Carrillo JE, Green AR, Betancourt JR. Cross-cultural primary care: a patient-based approach. *Ann Internal Med*. 1999 May 18; **130**(10): 829–34.

Centers for Disease Control and Prevention (CDC). Racial/ethnic disparities in prevalence, treatment, and control of hypertension: United States, 1999–2002. *MMWR Morbid Mortal Wkly Rep*. 2005 Jan 14; **54**(1): 7–9.

Chakraborty BM, Mueller WH, Reeves R, *et al*. For the patient. The importance of health behaviors for better heart health. Migration history, health behaviors, and cardiovascular disease risk factors in overweight Mexican-American women. *Ethn Dis*. 2003; **13**(1): 152.

Challis M. AMEE Medical Education Guide No. 11: portfolio-based learning and assessment in medical education. *Med Teach*. 1999; **21**: 370–86.

Chambers N. Close encounters: the use of critical reflective analysis as an evaluation tool in teaching and learning. *J Adv Nurs*. 1999; **29**(4): 950–7.

Charon R. Narrative medicine: a model for empathy, reflection, profession and trust. *JAMA*. 2001; **286**: 1897–1902.

Chisholm CD, Croskerry P. A case study in medical error: the use of the portfolio entry. *Acad Emerg Med*. 2004 Apr; **11**(4): 388–92.

Christiaens G, Baldwin JH. Use of dyadic role playing to increase student participation. *Nurse Educ*. 2002; **27**(6): 251–4.

Ciesielka DJ, Schumacher G, Conway A, *et al*. Implementing and evaluating a culturally-focused curriculum in a collaborative graduate nursing program. *Int J Nurs Educ Scholarsh*. 2005; **2**: Article 6.

Clark LT. Issues in minority health: atherosclerosis and coronary heart disease in African Americans. *Med Clin North Am*. 2005 Sep; **89**(5): 977–1001, 994.

Collins J. Education techniques for lifelong learning: giving a PowerPoint presentation: the art of communicating effectively. *Radiographics*. 2004 Jul–Aug; **24**(4): 1185–92.

Crandall SJ, George G, Marion GS, *et al*. Applying theory to the design of cultural competency training for medical students: a case study. *Acad Med*. 2003 Jun; **78**(6): 588–94.

Crisp C. The Gay Affirmative Practice Scale (GAP): a new measure for assessing cultural competence with gay and lesbian clients. *Soc Work*. 2006 Apr; **51**(2): 115–26.

Crosson JC, Deng W, Brazeau C, *et al*. Evaluating the effect of cultural competency training on medical student attitudes. *Fam Med*. 2004 Mar; **36**(3): 199–203.

Crystal S, Sambamoorthi U, Walkup JT, *et al*. Diagnosis and treatment of depression in the elderly Medicare population: predictors, disparities, and trends. *J Am Geriatr Soc*. 2003 Dec; **51**(12): 1718–28.

Culhane-Pera K, Like R, Lebensohn-Chialvo P, *et al*. Multicultural curricula in family practice residencies. *Fam Med*. 2000; **32**(3): 167–73.

DasGupta S, Meyer D, Calero-Breckheimer A, *et al*. Teaching cultural competency through narrative medicine: intersections of classroom and community. *Teach Learn Med*. 2006; **18**(1): 14–17.

Davis DA, Mazmanian PE, Fordis M, *et al*. Accuracy of physician self-assessment compared with observed measures of competence: a systematic review. *JAMA*. 2006 Sep 6; **296**(9): 1094–102.

Dolcourt JL, Zuckerman G. Unanticipated learning outcomes associated with commitment to change in continuing medical education. *J Cont Educ Health Prof*. 2003; **23**(3): 173–81.

Doorenbos AZ, Schim SM, Benkert R, *et al*. Psychometric evaluation of the cultural competence assessment instrument among healthcare providers. *Nurs Res*. 2005 Sep–Oct; **54**(5): 324–31.

Dovidio JF, Gaertner, SL, Kawakami, K., Hodson, G. Why can't we just get along? Interpersonal biases and interracial distrust. *Cultur Divers Ethnic Minor Psychol*. 2002; **8**(2): 88–102.

Dula A. The life and death of Miss Mildred: an elderly black woman. *Clin Geriatr Med*. 1994 Aug; **10**(3): 419–30.

Dunn AM. Culture competence and the primary care provider. *J Pediatr Health Care*. 2002 May–Jun; **16**(3): 105–11.

Eggert CH, West CP, Thomas KG. Impact of an audience response system. *Med Educ*. 2004 May; **38**(5): 576.

Eschbach K, Mahnken JD, Goodwin JS. Neighborhood composition and incidence of cancer among Hispanics in the United States. *Cancer*. 2005 Mar 1; **103**(5): 1036–44.

Eugenia E, Blanchard L. Action-oriented community diagnosis: a health education tool. *Int Q Commun Health Educ*. 1991; **11**(2): 93–110.

Exworthy M, Washington AE. Organizational strategies to tackle health-care disparities in the USA. *Health Serv Manag Res*. 2006 Feb; **19**(1): 44–51.

Ferguson WJ, Keller DM, Haley HL, *et al*. Developing culturally competent community faculty: a model program. *Acad Med*. 2003 Dec; **78**(12): 1221–8.

Fernandez A, Schillinger D, Grumbach K, *et al*. Physician language ability and cultural competence. An exploratory study of communication with Spanish-speaking patients. *J Gen Intern Med*. 2004 Feb; **19**(2): 167–74.

Flores G, Ngui E. Racial/ethnic disparities and patient safety. *Pediatr Clin North Am*. 2006 Dec; **53**(6): 1197–215.

Geuna S, Giacobini-Robecchi MG. The use of brainstorming for teaching human anatomy. *Anatomic Rec*. 2002 Oct 15; **269**(5): 214–16.

Gianakos D. Self-reflection, learning, and sharing mistakes. *Pharos Alpha Omega Alpha Honor Med Soc*. 1999; **62**(4): 33–4.

Glendon K, Ulrich D. Using games as a teaching strategy. *J Nurs Educ*. 2005 Jul; **44**(7): 338–9.

Goodyear-Smith F, Buetow S. Power issues in the doctor-patient relationship. *Health Care Anal*. 2001; **9**(4): 449–62.

Gordon J. Assessing students' personal and professional development using portfolios and interviews. *Med Educ*. 2003; **37**(4): 335–40.

Grant A, Dornan TL. What is a learning portfolio? *Diabet Med*. 2001; **18** (Suppl. 1): 1–4.

Grantmakers In Health. In the right words: addressing language and culture in providing health care. *Issue Brief (Grantmakers Health)*. 2003 Aug; **18**: 1–44.

Green AR, Miller E, Krupat E, *et al*. Designing and implementing a cultural competence OSCE: lessons learned from interviews with medical students. *Ethnic Dis*. 2007; **17**(2): 344–50.

Hall MJ, Adamo G, McCurry L, *et al*. Use of standardized patients to enhance a psychiatry clerkship. *Acad Med*. 2004; **79**: 28–31.

Hobgood C, Sawning S, Bowen J, *et al*. Teaching culturally appropriate care: a review of educational models and methods. *Acad Emerg Med*. 2006; **13**: 1288–95.

Hodges B, Regehr G, Martin D. Difficulties in recognizing one's own incompetence: novice physicians who are unskilled and unaware of it. *Acad Med*. 2001; **76**(Suppl.): S87–9.

Holt P. Challenges and strategies: weight management in type 2 diabetes. *Br J Commun Nurs*. 2006 Sep; **11**(9): 376–80.

Hook EB. Re: Neighborhood social environment and risk of death: multilevel evidence from the Alameda County study. *Am J Epidemiol*. 2000 Jun 1; **151**(11): 1132–3.

Horner RD, Salazar W, Geiger HJ, *et al*. Working Group on Changing Health Care Professionals' Behavior. Changing healthcare professionals' behaviors to eliminate disparities in healthcare: What do we know? How might we proceed? *Am J Manag Care*. 2004 Sep; **10** Spec No: SP12–19.

Johnson JT. Creating learner-centered classrooms: use of an audience response system in pediatric dentistry education. *J Dent Educ*. 2005 Mar; **69**(3): 378–81.

Johnson RL, Saha S, Arbelaez JJ, *et al*. Racial and ethnic differences in patient perceptions of bias and cultural competence in health care. *J Gen Intern Med*. 2004 Feb; **19**(2): 101–10.

Joyner B, Young L. Teaching medical students using role play: twelve tips for successful role plays. *Med Teach*. 2006 May; **28**(3): 225–9.

Kagawa-Singer M, Blackhall LJ. Negotiating cross-cultural issues at the end of life: "You got to go where he lives". *JAMA*. 2001 Dec 19; **286**(23): 2993–3001.

Kairys JA, Like RC. Caring for diverse populations: do academic family medicine practices have CLAS? *Fam Med*. 2006 Mar; **38**(3): 196–205.

Kamei R. Professionalism: looking for your blind spots. *Ann Acad Med Singapore*. 2006; **35**(12): 848–84.

Keppel K, Bilheimer L, Gurley L. Improving population health and reducing health care disparities. *Health Affairs*. 2007 Sep–Oct; **26**(5): 1281–92.

Kilbourne AM, Switzer G, Hyman K, *et al*. Advancing health disparities research within the health care system: a conceptual framework. *Am J Public Health*. 2006 Dec; **96**(12): 2113–21.

Kleinman A, Benson P. Anthropology in the clinic: the problem of cultural competency and how to fix it. *PLoS Med*. 2006 Oct; **3**(10): e294.

Kleinman A, Eisenberg L, Good B. Culture, illness, and care: clinical lessons from anthropologic and cross-cultural research. *Ann Intern Med*. 1978; **88**: 251–8.

Ko M, Heslin KC, Edelstein RA, *et al*. The role of medical education in reducing health care disparities: the first ten years of the UCLA/Drew Medical Education Program. *J Gen Intern Med*. 2007 May; **22**(5): 625–31.

Kobylarz FA, Heath JM, Like RC. The ETHNIC(S) mnemonic: a clinical tool for ethnogeriatric education. *J Am Geriatr Soc*. 2002 Sep; **50**(9): 1582–9.

Kripalani S, Bussey-Jones J, Katz MG, *et al*. A prescription for cultural competence in medical education. *J Gen Intern Med*. 2006 Oct; **21**(10): 1116–20.

Krueger PM, Neutens J, Bienstock J, *et al*. To the point: reviews in medical education teaching techniques. *Am J Obstet Gynecol*. 2004 Aug; **191**(2): 408–11.

Ladson GM, Lin JM, Flores A, *et al*. An assessment of cultural competence of first- and second-year medical students at a historically diverse medical school. *Am J Obstet Gynecol*. 2006 Nov; **195**(5): 1457–62.

Lambert SF, Brown TL, Phillips CM, *et al*. The relationship between perceptions of neighborhood characteristics and substance use among urban African American adolescents. *Am J Commun Psychol*. 2004 Dec; **34**(3–4): 205–18.

Larson L. Is your hospital culturally competent? (And what does that mean exactly?). *Trustee*. 2005 Feb; **58**(2): 20–3.

Lash TL, Fink AK. Re: "Neighborhood environment and loss of physical function in older adults: evidence from the Alameda County Study". *Am J Epidemiol*. 2003; **157**(5): 472–3.

Latessa R, Mouw D. Use of an audience response system to augment interactive learning. *Fam Med*. 2005 Jan; **37**(1): 12–14.

Latham CL, Fahey LJ. Novice to expert advanced practice nurse role transition: guided student self-reflection. *J Nurs Educ*. 2006 Jan; **45**(1): 46–8.

Latkin CA, Curry AD. Stressful neighborhoods and depression: a prospective study of the impact of neighborhood disorder. *J Health Soc Behav*. 2003; **44**(1): 34–44.

Lauderdale DS, Wen M, Jacobs EA, *et al*. Immigrant perceptions of discrimination in health care: the California Health Interview Survey 2003. *Med Care*. 2006 Oct; **44**(10): 914–20.

Lawson M, Nestel D, Jolly B. An e-portfolio in health professional education. *Med Educ*. 2004 May; **38**(5): 569–70.

Leventhal T, Brooks-Gunn J. Moving to opportunity: an experimental study of neighborhood effects on mental health. *Am J Public Health*. 2003 Sep; **93**(9): 1576–82.

Levin SJ, Like RC, Gottlieb JC. Useful clinical interviewing mnemonics. *Patient Care*. 2000; **34**: 189–90.

Lewis-Fernandez R, Diaz N. The cultural formulation: a method for assessing cultural factors affecting the clinical encounter. *Psychiatr Q*. 2002; **73**(4): 271–95.

Lie D, Boker J, Cleveland E. Using the tool for assessing cultural competence training (TACCT) to measure faculty and medical student perceptions of cultural competence instruction in the first three years of the curriculum. *Acad Med*. 2006 Jun; **81**(6): 557–64.

Like RC. Culturally competent family medicine: transforming clinical practice and ourselves. *Am Fam Physician*. 2005 Dec; **72**(11): 2189.

Lipson JG, DeSantis LA. Current approaches to integrating elements of cultural competence in nursing education. *J Transcultur Nurs*. 2007 Jan; **18**(1 Suppl.): 10S–20S; discussion 21S–27S.

Makoul G. Commentary: communication skills: how simulation training supplements experiential and humanist learning. *Acad Med*. 2006 Mar; **81**(3): 271–4.

McGarry K, Clarke J, Cyr MG. Enhancing residents' cultural competence through a lesbian and gay health curriculum. Acad Med. 2000 May; **75**(5): 515.

McKimm J, Jollie C, Cantillon P. ABC's of teaching and learning: web based learning. *BMJ*. 2003; **326**(7394): 870–3.

McMullan M, Endacott R, Gray MA, *et al*. Portfolios and assessment of competence: a review of the literature. *J Adv Nurs*. 2003; **41**(3): 283–94.

Melnyk BM, Small L, Morrison-Beedy D, *et al*. Mental health correlates of healthy lifestyle attitudes, beliefs, choices, and behaviors in overweight adolescents. *J Pediatr Health Care*. 2006 Nov–Dec; **20**(6): 401–6.

Menon AS, Moffett S, Enriquez M, *et al*. Audience response made easy: using personal digital assistants as a classroom polling tool. *J Am Med Inform Assoc*. 2004 May–Jun; **11**(3): 217–20.

Mihalic AP, Dobbie AE, Kinkade S. Cultural competence teaching in U.S. pediatric clerkships in 2006. *Acad Med*. 2007 Jun; **82**(6): 558–62.

Miller E, Green AR. Student reflections on learning cross-cultural skills through a 'cultural competence' OSCE. *Med Teach*. 2007 May; **29**(4): e76–84.

Miller RG, Ashar BH, Getz KJ. Evaluation of an audience response system for the continuing education of health professionals. *J Cont Educ Health Prof*. 2003; **23**(2): 109–15.

Morell VW, Sharp PC, Crandall SJ. Creating student awareness to improve cultural competence: creating the critical incident. *Med Teach*. 2002; **24**(5): 532–4.

Murray-Garcia JL, Harrell S, Garcia JA, *et al*. Self-reflection in multicultural training: be careful what you ask for. *Acad Med*. 2005 Jul; **80**(7): 694–701.

Narayan MC. The national standards for culturally and linguistically appropriate services in health care. *Care Manag J*. 2001–2002 Winter; **3**(2): 77–83.

Ngo-Metzger Q, Massagli MP, Clarridge BR, *et al*. Linguistic and cultural barriers to care. *J Gen Intern Med*. 2003 Jan; **18**(1): 44–52.

Nolinske T, Millis B. Cooperative learning as an approach to pedagogy. *Am J Occup Ther*. 1999 Jan–Feb; **53**(1): 31–40.

Nordstrom CK, Diez Roux AV, Jackson SA, *et al*. Cardiovascular Health Study. The association of personal and neighborhood socioeconomic indicators with subclinical cardiovascular disease in an elderly cohort. *Soc Sci Med*. 2004; **59**(10): 2139–47.

Nusbaum NJ. Health care disparities as a health care quality management challenge. *Health Care Manag*. 2007 Oct–Dec; **26**(4): 347–53.

O'Leary S, Diepenhorst L, Churley-Strom R, *et al*. Educational games in an obstetrics and gynecology core curriculum. *Am J Obstet Gynecol*. 2005 Nov; **193**(5): 1848–51.

Op't Holt TB. Problem-based and case-based learning in respiratory care education. *Respir Care Clin North Am*. 2005 Sep; **11**(3): 489–504.

Parbooshingh J. Learning portfolios: potential to assist health professionals with self-directed learning. *J Cont Educ*. 1996; **16**: 75–81.

Pena Dolhun E, Munoz C, Grumbach K. Cross-cultural education in U.S. medical schools: development of an assessment tool. *Acad Med*. 2003 Jun; **78**(6): 615–22.

Pickett KE, Ahern JE, Selvin S, *et al*. Neighborhood socioeconomic status, maternal race and preterm delivery: a case-control study. *Ann Epidemiol*. 2002 Aug; **12**(6): 410–8.

Pierce RO Jr. Ethnic and racial disparities in diagnosis, treatment, and follow-up care. *J Am Acad Orthopaed Surg*. 2007; **15** (Suppl. 1): S8–12.

Price EG, Beach MC, Gary TL, *et al*. A systematic review of the methodological rigor of studies evaluating cultural competence training of health professionals. *Acad Med*. 2005 Jun; **80**(6): 578–86.

Purnell L. The Purnell Model for cultural competence. *J Transcult Nurs*. 2002; **13**(3): 193–196.

Rabinowitz D, Melzer-Geva M, Ber R. Teaching the cultural dimensions of the patient-physician relationship: a novel approach using didactic trigger films. *Med Teach*. 2002 Mar; **24**(2): 181–5.

Rao SP, DiCarlo SE. Peer instruction improves performance on quizzes. *Adv Physiol Educ*. 2000 Dec; **24**(1): 51–5.

Regehr G, Hodges B, Tiberius R, *et al*. Measuring self assessment skills: an innovative relative ranking model. *Acad Med*. 1996; **71**(10 Suppl.): S52–S54.

Reilly JM, Ring J. Innovations in teaching: Turning point. *Fam Med*. 2003; **35**(7): 474–5.

Resnicow K, Davis R, Rollnick S. Motivational interviewing for pediatric obesity: conceptual issues and evidence review. *J Am Diet Assoc*. 2006 Dec; **106**(12): 2024–33.

Riley-Doucet C, Wilson S. A three-step method of self-reflection using reflective journal writing. *J Adv Nurs*. 1997; **25**(5): 964–8.

Ring, JM, The long and winding road: Personal reflections of an anti-racism trainer. Am J Orthopsychiatry, 2000; 70 (1): 73–81.

Rosa UW. Impact of cultural competence on medical care: where are we today? *Clinics Chest Med*. 2006 Sep; **27**(3): 395–9, v.

Rosen J, Spatz ES, Gaaserud AM, *et al*. New approach to developing cross-cultural communication skill. *Med Teach*. 2004 Mar; **26**(2): 126–32.

Rowland ML, Bean CY, Casamassimo PS. A snapshot of cultural competency education in US dental schools. *J Dent Educ*. 2006 Sep; **70**(9): 982–90.

Rust G, Kondwani K, Martinez R, *et al*. A crash-course in cultural competence. *Ethn Dis*. 2006; **16**(2 Suppl. 3): S3–29,36.

Rutledge CM, Garzon L, Scott M, *et al*. Using standardized patients to teach and evaluate nurse practitioner students on cultural competency. *Int J Nurs Educ Scholarsh*. 2004; **1**: Article17.

Schackow TE, Chavez M, Loya L, *et al*. Audience response system: effect on learning in family medicine residents. *Fam Med*. 2004 Jul–Aug; **36**(7): 496–504.

Schim SM, Doorenbos A, Benkert R, *et al*. Culturally congruent care: putting the puzzle together. *J Transcult Nurs*. 2007 Apr; **18**(2): 103–10.

Schim SM, Doorenbos AZ, Miller J, *et al*. Development of a cultural competence assessment instrument. *J Nurs Meas*. 2003 Spring–Summer; **11**(1): 29–40.

Schoonheim-Klein M, Walmsley, A. D, Habets, L, van der Velden, U. An implementation strategy for introducing an OSCE into a dental school. *Eur J Dent Educ*. 2005 Nov;9(4): 143–9

Schulman KA, Berlin JA, Harless W, *et al*. The effect of race and sex on physicians' recommendations for cardiac catheterization. *N Engl J Med*. 1999; **340**: 618–26.

Selig S, Tropiano E, Greene-Moton E. Teaching cultural competence to reduce health disparities. *Health Promot Pract*. 2006 Jul; **7**(3 Suppl.): 247S–55S.

Shapiro J, Hollingshead J, Morrison E. Self-perceived attitudes and skills of cultural competence: a comparison of family medicine and internal medicine residents. *Med Teach*. 2003 May; **25**(3): 327–9.

Shearer R, Davidhizar R. Using role play to develop cultural competence. *J Nurs Educ*. 2003 Jun; **42**(6): 273–276.

Siegel C, Haugland G. Chambers ED. Performance measures and their benchmarks for assessing organizational cultural competency in behavioral health care service delivery. *Admin Policy Mental Health*. 2003 Nov; **31**(2): 141–70.

Stafford F. The significance of de-roling and debriefing in training medical students using simulation to train medical students. *Med Educ*. 2005 Nov; **39**(11): 1083–5.

Stanhope V, Solomon P, Pernell-Arnold A, *et al*. Evaluating cultural competence among behavioral health professionals. *Psychiatr Rehab J*. 2005; **28**(3): 225–33.

Steinert Y. Student perceptions of effective small group teaching. *Med Educ*. 2004 Mar; **38**(3): 286–93.

Streeter JL, Rybicki FJ. A novel standard-compliant audience response system for medical education. *Radiographics*. 2006 Jul–Aug; **26**(4): 1243–9.

Suh EE. The model of cultural competence through an evolutionary concept analysis. *J Transcult Nurs*. 2004 Apr; 15(2): 93–102.

Tan MY. The relationship of health beliefs and complication prevention behaviors of Chinese individuals with type 2 diabetes mellitus. *Diabet Res Clin Pract*. 2004 Oct; **66**(1): 71–7.

Taylor SL, Lurie N. The role of culturally competent communication in reducing ethnic and racial healthcare disparities. *Am J Manag Care*. 2004 Sep; **10** Spec No: SP1–4.

Tervalon M, Murray-Garcia J. Cultural humility versus cultural competence: a critical distinction in defining physician training outcomes in multicultural education. *J Health Care Poor Underserved*. 1998; **9**(2): 117–25.

Thiel de Bocanegra H, Gany F. Good provider, good patient: changing behaviors to eliminate disparities in healthcare. *Am J Manag Care*. 2004 Sep; **10** Spec No: SP20–8.

Thom DH, Tirado MD, Woon TL, *et al.* Development and evaluation of a cultural competency training curriculum. *BMC Med Educ.* 2006; **6**: 38.

Thompson DR, Lachan R, Overpeck M, *et al.* School connectedness in the health behavior in school-aged children study: the role of student, school, and school neighborhood characteristics. *J School Health.* 2006 Sep; **76**(7): 379–86.

Thornton PL, Kieffer EC, Salabarria-Pena Y, *et al.* Weight, diet, and physical activity-related beliefs and practices among pregnant and postpartum Latino women: the role of social support. *Matern Child Health J.* 2006 Jan; **10**(1): 95–104.

Tiwari A, Tang C. From process to outcome: the effect of portfolio assessment on student learning. *Nurse Educ Today.* 2003; **23**(4): 269–77.

van Ryn M. Research on the provider contribution to the race/ethnicity disparities in medical care. *Med Care.* 2002; **40**(1 Suppl.): I140–51.

Vega WA. Higher stakes for cultural competence. *Gen Hosp Psychiatr.* 2005; **27**: 446–50.

Wakefield J, Herbert CP, Maclure M, *et al.* Commitment to change statements can predict actual change in practice. *J Cont Educ Health Prof.* 2003; **23**(2): 81–93.

Wakefield JG. Commitment to change: exploring its role in changing physician behavior through continuing education. *J Cont Educ Health Prof.* 2004; **24**(4): 197–204.

Wells MI. Beyond cultural competence: a model for individual and institutional cultural development. *J Commun Health Nurs.* 2000 Winter; **17**(4): 189–99.

White AA 3rd, Hill JA, Mackel AM, *et al.* The relevance of culturally competent care in orthopaedics to outcomes and health care disparities. *J Bone Joint Surg Am Vol.* 2007 Jun; **89**(6): 1379–84.

White AA 3rd, Hoffman HL. Culturally competent care education: overview and perspectives. *J Am Acad Orthopaed Surg.* 2007; **15** (Suppl. 1): S80–5.

White MI, Grzybowski S, Broudo M. Commitment to change instrument enhances program planning, implementation, and evaluation. *J Cont Educ Health Prof.* 2004; **24**(3): 153–62.

Willems S, Vanobbergen J, Martens L, *et al.* The independent impact of household- and neighborhood-based social determinants on early childhood caries: a cross-sectional study of inner-city children. *Fam Commun Health.* 2005 Apr–Jun; **28**(2): 168–75.

Williams RA. Cultural diversity, health care disparities, and cultural competency in American medicine. *J Am Acad Orthopaed Surg.* 2007; **15** (Suppl. 1): S52–8.

Winter RO, Birnberg BA. Teaching professionalism artfully. *Fam Med.* 2006 Mar; **38**(3): 169–71.

Yancy CW. The prevention of heart failure in minority communities and discrepancies in health care delivery systems. *Med Clin North Am.* 2004 Sep; **88**(5): 1347–68, xii–xiii.

Yen IH, Kaplan GA. Neighborhood social environment and risk of death: multilevel evidence from the Alameda County Study. *Am J Epidemiol.* 1999; **149**(10): 898–907.

Zamudio A, Hill K. Building closeness, understanding, and tolerance among residents: the family genogram. *Fam Med.* 2004; **36**(2): 625–6.

Other Resources

Clark A, Fong C, Jacobs MR. Health disparities among US women of color: an overview. Presented at the Institute of Women's Health Margaret E. Mahoney Annual Symposium: *Health Disparities Among Women of Color*; 2002 Apr 16; Washington, DC. Available from: www.jiwh.org

Los Angeles County Department of Health Services and the UCLA Center for Health Policy Research. *The Burden of Disease in Los Angeles County: A study of the patterns of morbidity and mortality in the county population.* Los Angeles: Los Angeles County Department of Health Services: UCLA Center for Health Policy Research; 2000.

National Standards for Culturally and Linguistically Appropriate Services in Health Care: Final Report. Rockville, MD: US Department of Health and Human Services, Office of Minority Health; 2001 Mar.